yoga and psychology

SUNY series in

Religious Studies

Harold Coward, editor

HAROLD COWARD

yoga and psychology

LANGUAGE, MEMORY, AND MYSTICISM

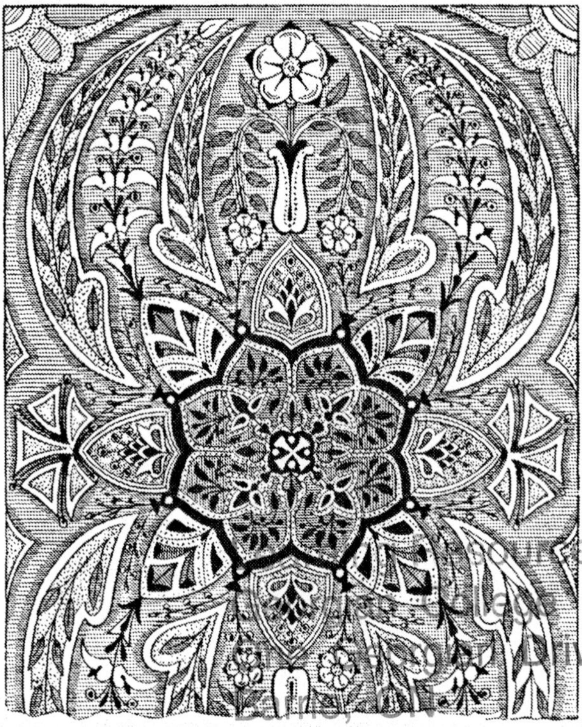

STATE UNIVERSITY OF NEW YORK PRESS

Published by
State University of New York Press
Albany

Printed in the United States of America

For information, address
State University of New York Press
90 State Street, Suite 700, Albany, NY 12207

Production, Laurie Searl
Marketing, Jennifer Giovani-Giovani

Library of Congress Cataloging-in-Publication Data

Coward, Harold G.
Yoga and psychology : language, memory, and mysticism / Harold Coward.
p. cm.—(SUNY series in religious studies)
Includes bibliographical references and index.
ISBN 0-7914-5499-1 (alk. paper) — ISBN 0-7914-5500-9 (pbk. : alk. paper)
1. Psychology and religion. 2. Yoga. 3. East and West. 4. Pataäjali. Yogasåtra. 5. Freud, Sigmund, 1856–1939. 6. Jung, C. G. (Carl Gustav), 1875–1961. I. Title. II. Series.

BF51 .C69 2002
181'.45—dc21

2002017732

10 9 8 7 6 5 4 3 2 1

to

PROFESSOR T. R. V. MURTI

contents

	Preface	ix
1	Introduction	1
	Part I Yoga and Language	
2	Āgama in the *Yoga Sūtras* of Patañjali	11
3	The Yoga Psychology Underlying Bhartṛhari's *Vākyapadīya*	21
4	Yoga in the *Vairāgya-Śataka* of Bhartṛhari	41
	Part II Yoga and Western Psychology	
5	Freud, Jung, and Yoga on Memory	51
6	Where Jung Draws the Line in His Acceptance of Patañjali's Yoga	61
7	Mysticism in Jung and Patañjali's Yoga	71
8	The Limits of Human Nature in Yoga and Transpersonal Psychology	83

preface

Patañjali's *Yoga Sūtras* (c. 200 CE), the classical statement of Eastern Yoga, are foundational for Hindu, Jaina, and Buddhist theology, philosophy, and spiritual practice. This book explores the fundamental contribution of Patañjali's *Yoga Sūtras* to the philosophy of language and theology of revelation of Bhartṛhari (c. 600 CE) in part I, and in part II analyzes where Western psychology (Freud, Jung, and Transpersonalists such as Washburn, Tart, and Ornstein) have been influenced by or reject Patañjali's Yoga. The part II analysis results in a key insight, namely, that there is a crucial difference between Eastern and Western thought with regard to how limited or perfectible human nature is—the West maintaining that we as humans are psychologically, philosophically, and theologically limited or flawed in nature and thus not perfectible, while Patañjali's Yoga (and Eastern thought generally) maintains the opposite. Indeed, for Yoga and the East, we will be reborn over and over until, through our yogic religious practice, we overcome our finite limitations, such as individual egos, and achieve union with the divine. Different Western responses to this Eastern claim are detailed in part II from complete rejection by Freud, Jung, and John Hick to varying degrees of acceptance by transpersonal psychologists such as Washburn, Tart, and Ornstein.

The lines of analysis in parts I and II have been gradually maturing over the past twenty years. The argument in part I that Patañjali's *Yoga Sūtras* were fundamental to Bhartṛhari's philosophy of language did not appear in my earlier books on that topic—*The Sphota Theory of Language*, Motilal Banarsidass, 1980, 1986, 1990, 1996, and *The Philosophy of the Grammarians*, Princeton University Press, 1990—because I was not completely sure of my scholarship on the point. My thinking was tested out in two early chapters of a 1976 Twayne book on Bhartṛhari that remained relatively obscure, circulating mainly among literature of India scholars. My thinking was further developed and tested in a 1985 article published in the *Indian Philosophical Quarterly*, which is little known outside India. As a result of feedback from these earlier publications and some revision, I am now confident of my scholarship on Patañjali's Yoga contributions to Bhartṛhari, which I have put together completely for the first time in part I. Chapters 3 and 4 are based on chapters 1 and 2 in my book *Bhartṛhari* © 1976 G.K. Hall.

In part II, my thinking on how Patañjali's Yoga has influenced Western psychology, and how a fundamental disagreement about human nature has appeared through that analysis, has developed and been tested in articles published in *Philosophy East and West*, a chapter from my SUNY book (*Jung and Eastern Thought*, 1985), and a new chapter on the transpersonal psychologists. All of this writing has been reworked a couple of times to highlight the major point of difference between Patañjali's Yoga and Western thinking on the limits of human nature—an insight which has only gradually clarified itself in my thinking but which I am now ready to engage fully. That this point, central to part II, is timely is evidenced by John Hick's most recent book, *The Fifth Dimension: An Exploration of the Spiritual Realm* (Oneworld, 1999) in which he devotes chapters 15 and 16 to dismissing Eastern claims of union with the divine as "metaphorical" rather than "literal" in nature. In my view, this is an unfair reductionism of Eastern claims, which are also shared by some Western mystics, by taking Kant's view of the limits of human nature and experience to be absolute. My position is that good comparative scholarship requires that we examine such claims within the presuppositions of their own worldviews, and that there is no "theological or philosophical helicopter" that will get us above all biases or presuppositions so as to determine which are absolute or right and which are wrong. Therefore, as scholars we must remain critical but open. It is this debate that is at the root of the disagreement as to the limits of human nature between Yoga and Western psychology, philosophy, and theology.

Taken together, parts I and II represent a culmination of my thinking on the significance of Patañjali's *Yoga Sūtras* over the past 25 years. It is the Yoga book I have wanted to write since I spent two years in Banaras (Varanasi) in 1972 and 1973, reading the *Yoga Sūtras* line by line in traditional guru-sishya style with my teacher, Professor T. R. V. Murti. (My book on Murti will appear in *The Builders of Indian Philosophy* series published by Manohar in 2002.)

I wish to thank Vicki Simmons for her assistance in the preparation of this book.

1

introduction

Yoga is a very popular word in the West these days. From exercise programs to meditation training, yoga teachers abound in most communities of Europe and North America. In bookstores the self-help sections contain numerous "yoga" titles. In most cases these modern presentations of yoga are updated versions of some aspect of the *Yoga Sūtras* of Patañjali, the basic presentation of the Indian Yoga school dating from 200 to 300 CE.[1] Among the classical schools of Indian philosophy, the Yoga school has been widely accepted as foundational as far as psychological processes are concerned. In this book we will show the role Yoga played in the classical Indian philosophy of language of Bhartṛhari, examine Yoga's influence on Carl Jung's psychology, observe parallels with Sigmund Freud's conception of how memory works, and study the impact of Yoga on transpersonal psychology. From a comparative perspective, it is noteworthy that during the past decades contemporary philosophy and psychology have refocused attention on "mind"[2] and "consciousness"[3]—topics that occupied the central focus in Yoga theory and practice. Thus the comparative explorations with Western psychology are timely.

YOGA IN INDIAN THOUGHT

Within Indian thought, conceptions such as *karma* (memory traces from previous actions or thoughts) and *saṁsāra* (rebirth) are taken as basic to all Jaina, Buddhist, and Hindu schools. So also there are certain common conceptions about the psychological processes of human nature (e.g., the existence of cognitive traces or *saṁskāras*) which are seen to exist in and through the specific differences of the various schools as a kind of commonly understood psychology. Jadunath Sinha supports this contention in his finding that the psychological conception of yogic intuition (*pratibhā*) is found in all schools with the exception of the Cārvāka and the Mīmāṁsā.[4] Mircea Eliade states that Yoga is one of the four basic motifs of all Indian thought. T. H. Stcherbatsky, the eminent Russian scholar of Buddhism, observes that Yogic trance (*samādhi*) and Yogic courses for the training of the mind in the achievement of *mokṣa* or *nirvāṇa* appear in virtually all Indian schools of thought.[5] Probably the most complete presentation of this traditional Indian psychology is to be found in the *Yoga Sūtras of Patañjali*, and it is from this source that the following overview is presented.[6]

Yoga starts with an analysis of ordinary experience. This is characterized by a sense of restlessness caused by the distracting influences of our desires. Peace and purity of mind come only when the distractability of our nature is controlled by the radical step of purging the passions. But if these troublesome passions are to be purged, they must be fully exposed to view. In this respect, Yoga predated Freud by several hundred years in the analysis of the unconscious. In the Yoga view, the sources of all our troubles are the karmic seeds (memory traces) of past actions or thoughts, heaped up in the unconscious, or storehouse consciousness, as it is called in Yoga, and tainted by ignorance, materialistic or sensuous desire, as well as the clinging to one's own ego. Thus, it is clear that traditional Yoga psychology gives ample recognition to the darker side of humans—the shadow consciousness.

At the ego-awareness level of consciousness, Yoga conceives of human cognition on various levels. There is the function of the mind in integrating and coordinating the input of sensory impressions and the resurgent memories of past thoughts and actions (*saṁskāras*). These may all be thought of as "learned" if we use behaviouristic terminology. Then there is the higher function of the mind in making discriminative decisions as to whether or not to act on the impulses that are constantly flooding one's awareness. This discriminative capacity (*buddhi*) is not learned but is an innate aspect of our psyche and has the capacity to reveal our true nature. This occurs when, by our discriminative choices, we negate and root out the polluting passions (*kliṣṭa karmas*) from our unconscious until it is totally purified of their distracting restlessness—their pulling and pushing of us in one direction and then another. Once this is achieved by disciplined self-effort, the level of egoic consciousness is transcended, since the notion of ego, I or me, is also ultimately unreal. It is simply a by-product of my selfish desiring. Once the latter is rooted out, the former by necessity also disappears, and the final level of human nature, pure or transcendent consciousness, is all that remains.

According to Yoga, transcendent consciousness is not immaterial but is composed of high-quality, high-energy luminous material (*sattvic citta*). Since all egoity has been overcome, there is no duality, no subject-object awareness, but only immediate intuition. All experience is transcendent of individuality, although this is described differently by the various schools of Indian thought. The Hindus, for example, overcome the subject-object duality by resolving all objectivity into an absolute subject (i.e., *Brahman*). The Buddhists seem to go in the opposite direction and do away with all subjectivity, leaving only bare objective experience (i.e., *Nirvāṇa*, which may be translated as "all ego and desiring is blown out"). For our present purpose, the metaphysical speculation, although interesting, is not important. What is significant is that Yoga psychology finds the essence of human nature to be at the transcendent level of consciousness, where ego and unconscious desires have been excised. The various kinds of Yogic meditation are simply different practical disciplines, or therapies, for removing conscious and unconscious desires, along with the accompanying ego-sense from the psyche.

Let us stay with Patañjali's *Yoga Sūtras*, although there are many other yogic schools of disciplined meditation from which one could choose (e.g., Tantric, Hatha, Jaina, Taoist, and Zen). For Patañjali there are five prerequisite practices and three ultimate practices. The prerequisite practices include: (1) self-restraints (*Yamas:* non-violence, truthfulness, non-stealing, celibacy, and absence of avarice) to get rid of bad habits; (2) good habits (*niyamas*) to be instilled (washing of body and mind, contentment with whatever comes, equanimity in the face of life's trials, study and chanting of scriptures, meditation upon the Lord); (3) body postures (*āsanas*) such as the lotus position to keep the body controlled and motionless during meditation; (4) controlled deepening of respiration (*prānāyāma*) to calm the mind; and (5) keeping senses (e.g., sight, hearing, and touch) from distracting one's mind (*pratyāhāra*) by focusing them on an object or point of meditation.

The ultimate practices are: (1) beginners spend brief periods of fixed concentration (*dhāraṇā*) upon an object (usually an image which represents an aspect of the divine that appeals to one, e.g., Īśvara, Śiva, Krishna, Kali); (2) as one becomes more expert, concentration upon the object is held for longer periods (*dhyāna*), and the sense of subject-object separation begins to disappear from one's perception; (3) *Samādhi* occurs when continuous meditation upon the object loses all sense of subject-object separation, and a state of direct intuition or becoming one with the object is achieved.

Through these yogic practices one has weakened the hold of the egocentric memories and desires (*karmas*) from the conscious and unconscious levels of one's psyche, and the discovery of the true self has begun. Four levels of *samādhi*, each more purified than the last, may be realized through repeated practice of yogic meditation. The final state (*nirvicāra samādhi*) occurs when all obstructing ego desires have been purged from the psyche, which is now like a perfectly clear window to the aspect of the divine (e.g., Īśvara, Śiva or, for a Westerner, perhaps Christ) which has served as the object of meditation. According to the *Yoga Sūtras*, any image will do. The divine image is only an instrument to aid in the direct experience of the transcendent, at which point the image is no longer needed.

Meditation of the sort prescribed by the *Yoga Sūtras* is esoteric in nature, requires the supervision of a teacher (*guru*) who has achieved perfection, and is a full-time occupation which, even in traditional India, was not possible for most people until the final stage of life in retirement from worldly affairs and withdrawal to a forest ashram. Another and much simpler yoga was and still is practiced by the masses—the yoga of the word. Thus the important inclusion in this book of Yoga's involvement with language. In Eastern psychology it is generally accepted that the chanting of a special scriptural word or phrase (*mantra*), chosen for one by one's teacher (*guru*), has power to remove the obstructing ego desires until the transcendent stands fully revealed.[7] The Yoga of the word assumes that the scriptural word and the divine are mutually intertwined, very much as stated in John's Gospel 1:1, "In the beginning was the Word, and the Word was with God, and the Word was God." The word is therefore filled with divine power and when meditated upon by repeated chanting is able to remove obstructions of consciousness. The *guru* chooses the scriptural word best suited to remove current obstructions (*karmas*) in the mind of the devotee. The power of the chosen *mantra* to remove obstructions is enhanced by the intensity and duration of the chanting. Chanting may be either aloud or silent. As the first obstructions are removed, the *guru* prescribes a new *mantra* better suited to tackle the remaining, more subtle obstructions. The more obstacles in the mind to be overcome, the more repetitions are needed. When the chanting removes the final obstacles, the psyche is like a purified or cleaned window fully revealing the divine as a direct intuition to the devotee; a vision of the lord is experienced, and *samādhi*, or union with the transcendent, is realized. With proper Yoga, words are experienced as having the power to remove ignorance (*avidyā*), reveal truth (*dharma*) and realize release or salvation (*mokṣa*). It is this traditional Eastern Yoga of the word that is behind the *mantra* chanting that is common throughout traditional Hinduism and Buddhism, and is today encountered in North America or Europe in the chanting of "Hare Krishna" and the teaching of meditation *mantras* by Transcendental Meditation. A detailed exploration of this practice is offered in part I.

Much of the current Western fascination for the East is with its much expanded view of human nature. This is what is felt to be lacking in contemporary Jewish and Christian religion. It is also this larger experience of human nature that is glimpsed in the psychedelic drug experience. The fascination of these practices is that they provide a technique which enables one to break out of the too-narrow Western rational-empirical view of human nature into which the whole society has been conditioned. But there are dangers here for the freeing of a person from his or her rigid ego encapsulation is only beneficial if the shadow or unconscious dimension of one's nature is also known and controlled. When this latter aspect is ignored, disastrous results occur. The person is "freed" from rational encapsulation, only to be made captive to the darker side of one's animal passions. The radically transcendent Eastern view of human nature is also open to the misinterpretation that "all is ONE" means nothing is good or evil, love equals hate, life equals death. The esoteric knowing of the transcendent mystical vision is open to dangerous distortion when placed in the hands of one who has not yet controlled the darker animal desires and power-hungry ego and who is not under the supervision of a *guru*.

Yoga's critique of modern life is that if the transcendent is not taken as absolute, then humankind is no longer seen as splendid or divine but simply "raw nature"—on par with minerals and rocks—to be manipulated for purposes of economic, political, and personal selfishness. First our lower nature must be controlled and our higher nature actualized, and then when the power of science and technology is placed in our hands, it will not enslave us in the endless attempt to satisfy our lower desires, as clearly has happened in the modern world.[8]

As usual, a middle road between the extremes seems indicated. A human being is neither all spiritual nor all animal desires, but a psychosomatic unity of the two. Two Western scholars attempt to champion such a balanced approach to psychology. Rudolf Otto argues for an analysis of humans which would include their feelings, rationality, and supra-rationality or transcendent consciousness.[9] Carl Jung is one modern Western thinker whose insights seem to be able to encompass most of the Yoga and Western psychologies without committing the academic sin of too much reductionism on one side or the other. Although a thoroughly Western psychologist, he is acclaimed by many from the East as expressing their understanding of human experience. The ways in which Jung has been influenced by Yoga, along with critical assessments of where he draws the line in his acceptance of Yoga are offered in part II, Yoga and Western Psychology.

Taken together, parts I and II offer an assessment of how the traditional Yoga psychology of India, as systematized by Patañjali in his *Yoga Sūtras*, supports the Indian view of how language functions and continues to influence modern Western thinkers such as Carl Jung and the Transpersonal Psychologists. A more detailed preview of each chapter follows.

OVERVIEW OF EACH CHAPTER

Chapter 2 examines the notion of *āgama* or how language functions as a valid communication of knowledge as presented in Patañjali's *Yoga Sūtras*. Not only our ordinary everyday encounter with language but more especially our experience of scripture is analyzed. How do we know that Hindu scripture, the Veda, is trustworthy? Because, says the *Yoga Sūtras*, it was spoken by the "Original Speaker," Īśvara, who is completely free from karmic obscuration and has directly "seen" the things spoken of in the Vedas. How this speech works is given detailed study. Īśvara, the seer/speaker of the Veda, at the beginning of each cycle of the cosmos, is described in the *Yoga Sūtras* as a uniquely pure *puruṣa*, untouched by obscuring *karma*, such as ignorance, egotistical desire, lust, hatred or clinging to life. Thus Īśvara has always been free and yet always in the world for the purpose of helping the rest of us to realize release from the cycle of *saṁsāra* (birth-death-rebirth). The chanting of Vedic verses or syllables (e.g., AUM) as *mantra* is a means by which language may function as a yoga to remove obscuring *karma* until it is all purged from consciousness and release is realized. The psychological mechanism by which such *mantra* chanting works to achieve release (*mokṣa*) is given detailed explanation in *Yoga Sūtras* I: 42–44 and is described in chapter 2.

In chapter 3 Patañjali's Yoga psychology is shown to be assumed by Bhartṛhari (c. 500 CE) in his *Vākyapadīya*, or Philosophy of Word and Sentence. The concepts outlined in *Yoga Sūtra* III: 17 are shown to provide the psychological processes necessary for Bhartṛhari's language theory to function in everyday life. And when it comes to the ultimate state of *mokṣa* or the realization of release, Patañjali's practices of *svādhyāya*, or concentrated study, including *mantra* chanting, provides the psychological mechanism by which that release (called by Bhartṛhari *śabdapūrvayoga*) may be achieved.

Just as Bhartṛhari's philosophy of language is shown to assume Patañjali's Yoga psychology, chapter 4 shows that Yoga psychology is also consistent with Bhartṛhari's poem the Vairāgya-Śataka. The five types of ordinary experience (*citta vṛtti*), identified by Patañjali in the *Yoga Sūtras* are given exposition in Bhartṛhari's poetry. In both the poem and in Yoga psychology, the *kleśas* or ordinary experiences of ignorance (*avidyā*), egoism (*asmitā*), passion (*rāga*), disgust (*dveṣa*), and clinging to life (*abhiniveśa*) are shown to end in suffering. The treatment offered by both Bhartṛhari and Patañjali is the renunciation of worldly desires by the concentration of *citta* or consciousness through Yoga. By intense devotional concentration on the Divine (Īśvara for Patañjali, Śiva for Bhartṛhari), release from rebirth may be realized.

Leaving India's traditional world of classical philosophy and psychology, we turn in part II to explicit influences or implicit parallels of Yoga in modern Western psychology. In chapter 5, parallels are noted between the Yoga conception of *karma* and the thinking of Freud and Jung on memory. It is suggested that Freud's theorizing and Eccles's experimentation on memory and motivation may well serve as the modern explanation of the neuro-physiological character of *karmic saṁskāras* and *vāsanās*—an explanation which, in Patañjali's time, involved a long discussion as to how the *guṇas*, or constituents of consciousness, function in various *karmic* states. In ancient Yoga, the storing of a memory trace was described as a latent deposit of *karma*, which would have as its neural basis a significant *tamas*, or physical structure component, perhaps parallel to the enlarged dendritic spines of modern neuro-physiology. The Yogic notion of *vāsanās*, or habit patterns, as resulting from repetitions of a particular memory trace, or *saṁskāra*, fits well with the modern idea of growth at the synaptic spines. Both Yoga and Freud agree that memory and motivation are parts of a single psychic process which also embodies choice or selection, but there is disagreement between Yoga and Freud as to the degree that this choice process is free or determined, as well as to the extent to which the processes of memory and motivation can be transcended. But both Yoga and Freud agree that the bulk of this memory/motivation psychological process occurs within the unconscious. Carl Jung seems to chart a middle course between Yoga and Freud. Although Jung remains resolutely Western and, along with Freud, denies that the unconscious could ever be totally overcome or transcended, Jung is influenced by the Yoga notion of *karma* in important ways. Jung read the *Yoga Sūtras*, and the notion of *karma* sparked the formation of Jung's archetype idea. Jung provides for collective memory and motivation from the unconscious in the form of the archetypes and allows for free choice in his requirement that the archetype be creatively developed by each individual within his or her own ego-consciousness. However, three differences between Jung and Yoga are identified, the most important being Jung's complete rejection of the Yoga contention that the ego-sense which memories produce is composed of nothing but obscuring *saṁskāras* (memory traces) and must be transcended for true knowledge and release (*mokṣa*).

Chapter 6 gives detailed explanations of the psychological processes of memory, perception, and knowledge offered by Patañjali's Yoga and Carl Jung's Analytical Psychology but focuses on the places where Jung draws the line in his acceptance of Yoga. While Jung was strongly influenced by Yoga psychology during the 1920s and 1930s, he is critical of the Yoga failure to distinguish adequately between philosophy and psychology. This, Jung argues, leads directly to Yoga intuition's over-reaching of itself, as, for example in the Yoga claim that the individual ego can be completely deconstructed and transcended and some form of universal consciousness achieved. For Jung, this claim is nothing more than the psychological projection of an idea which has no foundation in human experience. Yet this is precisely the Yoga claim, namely, that accomplished persons, such as the Buddha, had transcended the limitations of the individual ego and realized omniscience and release (*mokṣa*). However, according to Jung, to the extent that the removal of ego is achieved, the result would not be the recovery of memories from this and previous lives (the Yoga claim), but rather the person falling unconscious on the floor. This fundamental difference between Yoga and Jung in the assessment of the limits of human nature is explored in chapter 6 in terms of memory, perception, and knowledge.

Chapter 7 begins by defining mysticism so as to avoid current misinterpretations of mysticism as something "misty," vague, or emotional. By contrast, mystical experience has been experienced by the great mystics of all religions as something like sensory perception—only more direct and more vivid! For Patañjali's Yoga, mysticism is a case of intuition or supersensuous perception (*pratibhā*) from which distorting emotions have been purged by disciplined meditation. While modern Western philosophers such as Bertrand Russell have attempted to dismiss mysticism as merely subjective emotion, Patañjali's claim is just the opposite. According to his Yoga psychology, mystical experience is a case of the direct supersensuous perception of reality, with various levels of impurity of the mystical vision being caused by obscuring emotions not yet purged from the perception. In Yoga, the major cause of obscuring emotion is the individual ego (*ahamkāra*). The Yoga analysis achieves depths of sophistication beyond anything known in the West. Four levels of increasingly pure mystical experience when focused on an image (e.g., Īśvara, Krishna, Śiva) are identified, followed by the ultimate mystical experience, according to Patañjali, of imageless mystical experience—becoming one with the divine that is beyond or behind the image or object. For this to happen, the limiting individual ego has to be totally transcended, and that indeed is the goal of Patañjali's Yoga practice. While Carl Jung, in his analysis of mystical experience, also begins with an object (e.g., a cross) as the point of focus for individuation of the unconscious archetype into a conscious symbol, Jung differs from Yoga in that he never leaves the object or the experiencing ego. This difference, which is explored in chapter 7, is profound for its implication as to whether mystical experience is a full and "literal" experience of the divine, or "metaphorical," as John Hick suggests in his most recent book.[10] It is also important for an assessment as to the limits of human nature: can we as humans be perfected or actualized beyond the finite ego limits accepted by most Western philosophy, psychology, and theology?[11]

Chapter 8 continues this discussion as to the different assessment of the limits of human nature in Yoga when compared with modern Western thought, especially the transpersonal psychologists. Like Jung, Michael Washburn is shown to attempt to bridge Eastern and Western thought. While Washburn goes further than the structural-hierarchial paradigms of Piaget and Kohlberg and simplifies Freud's Id, Ego, and Superego, Washburn, like Jung before him, remains resolutely Western in his claim that the limitations of ego-awareness can never be totally transcended, as Yoga psychology claims. Alan Roland, a New York psychiatrist, goes further in the Yoga direction by adding a psycho-social analysis showing that Indians living in extended families have an extended sense of self, a "we-self" as he calls it, in contrast to the limited "I-self" of modern Western experience. This "we-self" has permeable boundaries and is open to expansion outward to include both nature and the divine, much as Patañjali's Yoga suggests. The chapter concludes with a consideration of the argument by the contemporary Western philosopher John Hick for the necessity of an ego-limited human nature, even in mystical experience, in contrast to the more open approach of transpersonal psychologists such as Charles Tart or Robert Ornstein.

Part I

yoga and language

2

Āgama in the *Yoga Sūtras* of Patañjali

As humans, we live and move and have our being in our use of words. Although animals can use signs and sounds to signal one another, it would seem that humanity alone possesses the ability to think and speak, and at the same time to be aware of what he or she is thinking and speaking. Aristotle established the classical Western conception of humanity as the beings who have language (*logos*). Even to criticize its limitations, sometimes to the extent of negating it, we have to use language. When a speaker makes use of words to convey the meaning of something not present on the scene, and when this is understood by the hearer, language functions. Today the question being asked is, "How neutral or unbiased is the word communication process?" In modern thought, both structuralism and feminism see word use in the past to be an alien system weighing down human consciousness. For many today it seems that the comfortable "dwelling house of language" has become Nietzsche's "prison-house of language."[1] Implicit in all of this is a return to the awareness of language as power—power to obscure or to reveal.

The obscuring or revealing power of words was well recognized in the Indian speculations upon language. Indeed the major *āstika/nāstika* (Orthodox, saying "yes to the Vedas"/Heteradox, saying "no to the Vedas") division of the schools of Indian philosophy is predicated upon the degree of revealing power allowed to words, particularly the words of the Veda. Thus an essential point of focus for the study of any school of thought is: "How do ordinary words and the special scriptural words reveal or obscure reality?" Implied within that question is the further, and perhaps more crucial, question, "Is the revealing power of words a way of salvation or release?" The focus of this chapter is upon the way in which these two questions are answered in Patañjali's *Yoga Sūtra*.[2] To begin, the *Yoga Sūtra's* analysis of the revealing (and obscuring) power of ordinary words will be examined. Next the special spiritual power of Īśvara's words (scriptural words) will be studied. This second aspect of language is of special interest, as the *Yoga Sūtras* are not usually thought of as championing scripture, or meditation upon scripture, as a way of release. However, in the wake of attention being given to the Vivaraṇa sub-commentary (attributed to Śaṅkara) on the Vyāsa-bhāṣya[3] and to Gerald Larson's suggestion that the core of Śaṅkara's teaching is really a Vedāntinization of Sāṁkhya-Yoga,[4] an accurate assessment is needed of the role of word and scripture (*āgama*) in the *Yoga Sūtras* and its commentaries.

THE POWER OF ORDINARY WORDS

Does ordinary or everyday word-use reveal or obscure reality? Do such words convey knowledge? These questions are addressed in *Yoga Sūtras* I: 7. *Sūtra* I: 7 identifies verbal communication (*āgama*), along with perception (*pratyakṣa*) and inference (*anumāna*), as sources of valid knowledge (*pramāṇa*). *Āgama* is defined by Vyāsa in his commentary as follows:

> An object perceived or inferred by a competent [trustworthy, *āpta*] man is described by him in words with the intention of transferring his knowledge to another. The mental modification which has for its sphere the meaning of words is the verbal cognition to the hearer. When the speaker has neither perceived nor inferred the object, and speaks of things which cannot be believed, the authority of Verbal Cognition fails. But it does not fail in the original speaker [Īśvara] with reference to either the object of perception or of inference.[5]

The essential aspects of this definition are repeated again by Vyāsa in his discussion of truthfulness as one of the *Yamas* described in *Yoga Sūtra* II: 29.

> Veracity consists in thought and word being in accord with facts. Speech and mind corresponds to what has been seen, heard and inferred as such. Speech is uttered for the purpose of transferring one's knowledge to another. It can only be said to have been employed for the good of others and not for their injury, if it is not deceptive, confused or barren in knowledge.[6]

The answer of Patañjali and Vyāsa to the question, "Do ordinary or everyday words convey knowledge?" is clear. Words convey knowledge if they are true and not deceptive or confused. This requires that the speaker have a purified mind, a mind that does not selfishly twist in the telling of what has been seen or inferred, a mind cleansed of karmic obscuration. Such a mind is found in a trustworthy or competent person (*āpta*). When a clear-minded person speaks of something that has been seen or inferred, that knowledge is transferred via the hearing of the spoken word to the mind of the listener, and verbal communication (*āgama*) has taken place. Vācaspati Miśra points out in his gloss that the essential requirement for *āgama* to take place is that the speaker be an *āpta*—a competent, trustworthy person, one who has clear comprehension of the other two *pramāṇas*, or means of valid knowledge (perception and inference), as well as being skilled and compassionate in the passing on of knowledge.[7] All of this is clearly exemplified in the case of a true teacher. To succeed in *āgama*, or verbal communication, the teacher must perceive reality (the object) clearly (*pratyakṣa*) or reason (*anumāna*) about reality without confusion, and then pass on the knowledge so obtained with compassion for the student without any twisting for the purposes of personal fame or fortune. Such a teacher is *āpta*, or competent and trustworthy. Such teaching is *āgama*, or the verbal communication of valid knowledge. The teaching or verbal communication may still fail if the mind of the hearer is too covered with karmic impurity or too distracted to pay attention. This would seem to be the reason for the restriction of Vedic study to the upper three castes—to those who have purified their minds sufficiently to meet the entrance requirement for becoming a student.

In the gloss on Vyāsa's commentary attributed to Śaṅkara, the author stresses that the authority ascribed to *āgama* is normally to be understood with reference to the hearer rather than the speaker. For the hearer, the authoritativeness of the knowledge arises not from a direct perception of the object or from inference, since these cognitions took place in the mind of the speaker. Authority, for the hearer, is thus vested in the trustworthiness of the speaker. Authority comes into *āgama* on the side of the hearer, who has to accept the knowledge of the speaker as authoritative since he has not had the first-hand experience of perception or inference.[8] For the speaker, by contrast, the authority of the knowledge rests not with the process of verbal transmission (*āgama*), but with his prior experience of perception or inference, the original experience which his words report. Here provision is made in Vyāsa's commentary for the identification of unauthoritative or invalid *āgama*: "When the speaker has neither perceived nor inferred the object, and speaks of things which cannot be believed, the authority of *āgama* fails."[9] Vācaspati offers an example: "These ten pomegranates will become six cakes." This incredible thing, which the speaker has neither seen nor inferred, produces a verbal communication that, as J. H. Woods puts it, "wavers."[10] The question is then raised in Vācaspati's gloss, "If that be so, then the verbal communication even of such persons as Manu would waver [and thus not be authoritative], for even they declared things which they themselves had not seen or inferred."[11] Manu is rescued, however, by the answer that since he only says what is in the Veda, what he says is trustworthy because the Veda is trustworthy. How do we know that the Veda is trustworthy and authoritative? We know so, says Vācaspati, because it was spoken by the Original Speaker, Īśvara, who himself had directly seen or inferred the things spoken in the Vedas.

At this point in the discussion the commentaries raise the question of the validity of the metaphysical knowledge of the Veda. Although the description of *āgama* offered in I: 7 may be acceptable as far as knowledge from everyday word-use is concerned, it seems to break down when related to the metaphysical knowledge which the *Ṛṣis* of the Vedas and sages such as Manu claim to convey. For the moment this problem is summarily answered by invoking Īśvara as the Original Speaker who was omniscient and therefore of unquestionable authority. But later in the *Yoga Sūtras* a detailed explanation as to how this is the case is offered.

As a postscript to our discussion of *Yoga Sūtra* I: 7, it is of interest to note that in his commentary Śaṅkara argues that analogy (*upamāna*) presupposes words and therefore is not a separate *pramāṇa* (as Vedāntins claim) but a sub-case of *āgama*.[12] This interpretation is noteworthy on two counts. First, it shows Śaṅkara being true to the

Indian scholarly tradition, by which to be judged a good scholar one must be able to exegete an opponent's position with such skill that the result is accepted by the opponent as a valid contribution to his own thought. To do so in this passage, Śaṅkara has to go against his own Advaita Vedānta position, which treats *upmāna* as an independent *pramāṇa*. The second aspect of interest is that those who deny *upmāna* usually absorb it under inference, not *āgama* as Śaṅkara has done.

On a quite different note, Swami Hariharānanda Āraṇya suggests that mental telepathy involves thought transference and thus ought to be understood as a special case of verbal communication (*āgama*). How is this so? Some persons, he suggests, are specially gifted with the power to find out what is in another mind or to communicate one's own thought to another. Such persons are "mind-readers" and possess the power of thought-transference or telepathy. He offers the following example:

> If you think that a book is in such and such a place, that thought will at once rise in their mind, i.e., they will come to have a knowledge of the existence of the book in that place. How does the cognition come to the thought-readers? Not by direct perception. The words uttered mentally by one person and the sure knowledge arising out of their meaning affects the other mind and produces similar knowledge in that mind.[13]

Such a cognition, says Āraṇya, is certainly not from either direct perception or inference. It must therefore be a special case of verbal communication (*āgama*) in which the words are mentally spoken but not uttered aloud, and a purified mind "sees" them and thus receives the knowledge contained in the thought but unspoken sentence.

THE POWER OF SCRIPTURAL WORDS

How is it that the scriptural words of the Veda, invoked by the *Ṛṣis* and sages, reveal reality? Since the objects of scriptural words are metaphysical (i.e. they cannot be seen or inferred), how can such words be trusted as *āgama*, or valid verbal knowledge? Do such words have the power to effect release? These questions are taken up in *Yoga Sūtras* I: 24–29.

We recall that in *Yoga Sūtra* I: 7 the question was raised as to how the words of sages such as Manu could be judged as *āgama*, or authoritative, since they spoke of metaphysical things which they had neither seen nor inferred. The quick answer given in the commentaries on I: 7 was that words of Manu and the sages were trustworthy in that they merely repeated the words of the Veda which had been directly seen by the original speaker Īśvara. *Yoga Sūtras* I: 24–29 examine this answer in detail. As we analyze *Yoga Sūtra* I: 24–29, Śaṅkara's Vivaraṇa gloss on the Vyāsa bhāṣya will be given special attention, as it is in Śaṅkara's treatment of Īśvara and the Vedas, that "the Vedāntinizing of Sāṇkhya-Yoga" suggested by Gerald Larson should be most evident. Larson's suggestion needs careful assessment as it would change current thinking, which sees Śaṅkara's philosophy as a direct descendant of Mīmāṁsā and/or Buddhist thought, to instead seeing Śaṅkara as a direct descendant of Sāṇkhya-Yoga.

In *Yoga Sūtra* I: 24 the so-called Original Speaker, Īśvara, is defined as a special kind of self or *puruṣa* which is beginninglessly untouched by the taints of *karmas*, or their fruition, or their latent impulses (*vāsanā*). The taints or hindrances, of which Īśvara is free, include ignorance, ego-sense, desire, hatred, and clinging to life. Īśvara has never been touched by any such experiences and thus is a unique *puruṣa*. While all other *puruṣas* have to break their bonds with such experiences to realize release, Īśvara has always been and always will be free. Yet he is at the same time in the world, in *prakṛti*, because, as Vyāsa puts it, he has assumed a body of pure *sattva* (transparent consciousness). It is this pure sattvic body which enables Īśvara to function as a mind in the world. Vācaspati Miśra notes that Īśvara takes on this pure *sattva* body due to this wish to help those *puruṣas* still in bondage. Unlike others whose *sattva* is tainted by admixtures of *rajas* and *tamas*, Īśvara's *sattva* is free of other *guṇas* (obscuring qualities of consciousness), and this enables him to be in the world yet untouched by it. Vācaspati offers the analogy of the actor who takes on the role of Rama and yet does not confuse his identity as *puruṣa* with that of the worldly *prakṛti*. In answer to the question as to what causes Īśvara to take on this *sattva* body, the answer is given by Vācaspati that at the end of each cycle of creation Īśvara thinks to himself, "after this period of latency finishes I must again assume a pure *sattva* body so as to continue to help the world." This thought lays down a seed or memory trace which causes Īśvara to take on a *sattva* body at the start of the next creation cycle. Again Vācaspati offers an analogy. Īśvara's action between the cycles of creation is like that of Chaitra, who contemplates, "Tomorrow I must get up at day-break," and then having slept gets up at that very time because of a *vāsanā*, or habitual memory trace, laid down by his contemplation.[14]

In answer to the question, "what is the function of this *sattva* body that Īśvara takes on at the start of each new creation cycle?" Vyāsa replies that its function is to reveal the scriptures. Indeed, in response to an opponent who asks for proof of the existence of Īśvara's special *sattva* body, the existence of the scriptures are cited. Furthermore, the authority of the scriptures comes from the fact that they are a manifestation of Īśvara's *sattva*. Clearly this argument is circular, and Vyāsa admits that there is a beginningless relation between the scriptures, with their authority on spiritual matters, and Īśvara's *sattva* body. This is the presupposition upon which the *Yoga Sūtra* definition of the authority of *āgama*, with regard to supersensuous matters, is grounded. In his comment on Vyāsa, Śaṅkara takes the further step of arguing that all of this is established by inference as follows: because Īśvara's *sattva* body has never been tainted, it is unique and therefore unsurpassed by any other power; all others have been tainted. Thus the special *sattva* of Īśvara and the scriptures it reveals can never be equalled. "Therefore this Lord is one whose power has none to equal or surpass it, and it is established that the Lord is a special Puruṣa apart from *pradhāna* and other *Puruṣas*."[15]

Having established the existence of Īśvara's special *sattva* body on the basis of testimony and inference, *Yoga Sūtra* I: 25 goes on to examine its special quality of omniscience. Unlike our minds, in which the proportion of *tamas* (dullness of consciousness) that is present prevents us from knowing supersensuous things, and thus restricts our use of *āgama* to words based on inference and sensuous perception, Īśvara's pure *sattva* reflects all of reality, including both the sensuous and the supersensuous: "All certain knowledge, of past or future or present or a combination of them, or from extra-sensory perception, whether that knowledge be small or great, is the seed of [Īśvara's] omniscience."[16] The characterization of this omniscient knowledge in Īśvara's *sattva* is a "seed" (*bija*) is consistent with the idea that it "sprouts" or manifests itself anew in the Vedas at the start of each cycle of creation. Out of all the *puruṣas*, only Īśvara has the power to fulfill this crucial role beginninglessly, since only he has a *sattva* which has never been tainted by *karma*. The great saints such as the Buddhas or Jainas were all at one stage immersed in *karma*, and due to that limitation do not have the same fullness of omniscience as Īśvara, since he has never been limited by *karma*. Thus, as Patañjali says, Īśvara is the most perfect *puruṣa* in whom the seed of omniscience is at its utmost limit or excellence (*Yoga Sūtra* I: 25).

In his commentary Śaṅkara adds some helpful examples. By virtue of his pure *sattva* body, which is free of the limitations, such as senses like the eye, that constrain the rest of us, Īśvara is in simultaneous contact with every object and so can perceive everything. For example, says Śaṅkara, if a light is set inside a clay jar with holes in it, its light will illumine only what is directly outside of the holes. But this same light, when its covering jar has been shattered, illumines everything without being dependent on the holes for a path. Just so, the *sattva* body of Īśvara, being beginninglessly untouched by any covering *karma*, has perception of absolutely everything at the same time.[17] Thus the superiority of Īśvara's knowledge over the knowledge of all others.

In passing it might be noted that Śaṅkara finds himself quite at home with the description of Īśvara put forth in this *sūtra*. Indeed the stress on the unlimited nature of Īśvara leads smoothly into Śaṅkara's Advaita Vedānta notion of Brahman. Indeed, Śaṅkara, in answering an opponent who claims that Īśvara must perceive nothing because of his lack of sense organs, says that if the opponent insists on understanding perception through limitations or sense organs, he could think of Īśvara as experiencing "everything through the sense organs of all living beings, into which the inmost self, itself without sense organs, has entered as into a house."[18] Suddenly the Advaita Vedānta notion of *saguṇa* qualified Brahman has appeared. The only change required was to universalize Īśvara so as to absorb all other *puruṣas*, making Īśvara into the inmost self, the *Ātman*. By focusing on the omniscience of Īśvara, we see the ease with which Śaṅkara could, as Larson suggests, Vedāntinize the *Yoga Sūtras*.

The last part of Vyāsa's commentary of *Yoga Sūtra* I: 25 emphasizes the motivation of Īśvara—to help the persons caught in the whirling vortext of *saṁsāra*. Since the motivation is for others and not for himself, Īśvara remains free from the taint of *karma*. His freely chosen purpose, as explained in *Yoga Sūtra* I: 26, is to give help by teaching knowledge and *dharma*. In doing this, Īśvara is the first or original speaker who may be thought of as dictating the Vedas to the *Ṛṣis* at the start of each creation cycle. Because the words of the Vedas are based on the direct (but supersensuous) perception of Īśvara, they qualify as *āgama*—the special *āgama* that gives valid knowledge of extra-sensory or divine reality. Vācaspati in his gloss on I: 25 defines *āgama* as including *śrutri* (the Vedas) and *smṛti* (the Epics and Purāṇas). The *āgama*, or scripture, is characterized as that from which the spiritual means for worldly happiness and final bliss come to one's mind. From this scripture also comes information about Īśvara, such as his name and his special qualities. Śaṅkara, in his commentary on I: 26 points out that the expression "first knower or speaker" should not lead us to think of Īśvara in terms of an absolute beginning. Rather "first" or "original" expresses that fact that Īśvara is not limited or particularized by time. He has always been there. And since the Vedas have a beginningless relation with Īśvara's *sattva*, they too have always been there. However, the *Ṛṣis* and other sages are limited by time.

Having established the eternality of Īśvara and of his speaking of the Vedas as valid *āgama*, the way is now cleared for the final question to be answered: "Do these Vedic words, now seen to be valid knowledge (*āgama*), also enable one to realize release?" To answer this question, *Yoga Sūtras* I: 27–29 may be taken together. In his gloss on *Yoga Sūtra* I: 23 Vācaspati Miśra states that by devotion of mind, speech, and body to Īśvara, release may be realized. Later in the text, when the *angas*, or aids to yoga, are being discussed, the contention is again stated: by devoting all actions to Īśvara with no thought for oneself, one is freed from doubts (*vitarka*) and the seed of rebirth is destroyed (*Yoga Sūtra* II: 32). How does one perform such devotion to Īśvara? *Sūtras* I: 27 and 28 give us the answer. In I: 27 we are taught that *AUM*, the *praṇava* or sacred word, connotes Īśvara, and in I: 28 that by the devotional chanting (*japa*) of *AUM* release may be realized.

Śaṅkara, commenting on I: 26, observes that devotion upon things which cannot be known directly (i.e., by perception or inference) is to be done through the medium of the word. It is Īśvara who is expressed by the word *AUM*; the sound of the word evokes its meaning. The theory of language implied here is given detailed analysis later in the text under *Yoga Sūtra* III: 19. The relationship between word and meaning is shown to be eternal and grounded in the *sphoṭa* or meaningful illumination of Īśvara's sāttvic consciousness. It is worth noting in passing that the theory of language assumed in the *Yoga Sūtras* is consistent with the views of the Grammarians found in Patañjali's *Mahābhaṣya* and Bhartṛhari's *Vākyapadīya*.[19]

An opponent raises the question, does the ability of *AUM* to evoke Īśvara arise from conventional usage or is it something fixed like the relation between a lamp and its light? The intent of the question is to suggest that a convention is involved and that the word *AUM* should not be seen as *necessarily* evoking Īśvara; *AUM* could just as well be related to another name such as Śiva. Vyāsa responds that the relationship between Īśvara and the word *AUM* is fixed like that between a lamp and its light. So even at first hearing, Īśvara is evoked, just as the sun is evoked by its light. Conventional or ordinary usages only direct attention to that relationship between *AUM* and Īśvara which has existed beginninglessly. It is like the relationship of father and son which is inherently fixed, but which is made clear by conventional usage of words such as "He is that man's father" or "That man is his son." The conventional usage of words serves only to reveal the fixed relations and meanings that have permanently existed. Śaṅkara's gloss effectively summarizes the meaning of Patañjali's *sūtra* and Vyāsa's commentary.

> If there were not the fixed relation between this expressive word and what it expresses, it would not be true that through the form of *praṇava*, *Om*, the Lord [Īśvara] is met face to face . . . But since there is a fixed relation between this expression and what it expresses, it is proper to employ *Om* as a means for practising worship of God [Īśvara], and this is the purport of the whole commentary.[20]

Having recognized the power of *AUM* to reveal Īśvara, the yogin in sūtra I: 28 is directed to repeat it and meditate upon its meaning. From the perspective of modern secular consciousness, it is easy for us to miss the depth of meaning implied in this *sūtra*. The modern mind, unacquainted with the subtleties of yogic concentration, probably envisages the simple-minded chanting of the *mantra* by a devotee with a rosary in hand. The thought that such a primitive ritual could lead to a full revelation of the Lord is likely to be quickly dismissed as meaningless and empty ritual. Witness, for example, the judgement of Friedrich Heiler in his modern classic on the history and psychology of prayer. Ritual devotional prayer, he concludes, is no longer a free outpouring of the heart: "It becomes a fixed formula which people recite without feeling or mood of devotion, untouched both in heart and mind."[21] Contrary to such a simple-minded misconception of what is implied, *Yoga Sūtra* I: 28 specifies that the chanting of *AUM* with deep yogic concentration brings not only the full meaning of Īśvara to mind, but takes one beyond even that to a direct supersensory, "face-to-face" encounter. The psychological process by which this takes place is spelled out in detail in *Yoga Sūtras* I: 42–44. What Vyāsa describes under I: 28 as coming to ***know well*** the relation between the word, *AUM*, and its meaning, Īśvara, through constant repetition and habituation of the mind, is given technical analysis in the later passage. Four stages of increasingly pure habituation of the mind are described. In *Yoga Sūtra* I: 42 the lowest and most impure level is that in which the chanting of *AUM* evokes an experience of its object, Īśvara, which is mixed up by the conventional usage of the word and the meanings (*artha*) that the conventional usages have signified (e.g., Īśvara as "God," "Lord," "Master Yogi," or even Eliade's "macroyogin").[22] This is the *savitarkā samādhi* experience of *AUM* (and its supersensuous object Īśvara), and to reach even this level considerable study and practice is presupposed. The mixing up or distortion (*vikalpa*) that the chanting of *AUM* is evoking in our minds at that stage results from the habitual way in which we have used the *mantra* in this and previous lives and the meanings (theological and otherwise) we have been conditioned by convention to attach to it. Such conditional cognitions are either accepted from the traditional systems of thought or may be made up by one's own imaginative thinking. For example, this would seem to be what is happening when Śaṅkara interprets the Īśvara of Yoga in such way as to appear co-extensive with the Brahman of Advaita Vedānta. Thus at this lowest level of *samādhi*, or devotional meditation, even when we manage to block out external distractions and concentrate our minds sufficiently so as to become "caught up into oneness" with the *praṇava* (*AUM*), the *samādhi* achieved, although manifesting Īśvara, is obscured and distorted by our habitual way of speaking and thinking.

As one continues to concentrate only on the *praṇava*, through chanting the force of the habitual accretions is weakened (through non-fruition) until such karmic seeds exhaust themselves and disappear from the mind. One's chanting of *AUM* now evokes only its natural and eternal reference, Īśvara. As Vyāsa puts it in his commentary on I: 42, only then is the *sattva* aspect of the devotee's consciousness freed from the *rajas* or emotional obscuration so that the object (Īśvara, in this case) makes its appearance in the mind in its own distinct nature. This is the *nirvitarka samādhi* of Īśvara. From the reports of yogis like Vyāsa on I: 24, in this experience one comes to know Īśvara as the original speaker of the Vedas to the *Ṛṣis*, although, of course, to put this into conventional words, as we have just done, already reduces us back to the level of *savitarka*. To know it in its *nirvitarka* purity, one must experience it for oneself.

The third level of *savicāra samādhi* is reached through yet more repetition of the chant and is described in *Yoga Sūtra* I: 43. Śaṅkara suggests, in his comment on this *sūtra*, that at this stage the devotee should be repeating *AUM* mentally rather than aloud. At the *savicāra* level one "perceives" Īśvara's pure *sattva* body. In *savicāra* experience the flow of consciousness so completely identifies with the object (Īśvara) alone that the devotee's mind is, as it were, devoid of its own nature. I take Vyāsa to mean by this that there is a complete loss of ego-consciousness. This does not mean that one lapses into some sort of stupor, as Jung insists on maintaining.[23] On the contrary, what is implied is that one is so "caught up" into Īśvara that there is no room left for a separate awareness of one's own ego as the thing that is having the experience. One has forgotten oneself. Īśvara, in all its vividness of external characteristics (the *praṇava* "sprouting" into the Vedas) and internal qualities (a pure *sattva* body), totally commands one's attention. The only distinguishing characteristics are provided by the object (Īśvara) itself. The devotee's knowledge ("knowing by becoming one with Īśvara") is complete, but it is knowledge only of the present moment in space and time.

The final stage of *nirvicāra samādhi* differs from the *savicāra* stage in that in the *nirvicāra* the limitation to the present moment in time and space is overcome (*Yoga Sūtra* I: 44). Now the devotee is so completely one with Īśvara that Īśvara's relationship with the *praṇava* and the Vedas (of which it is the seed) is seen to have existed in all previous cycles (beginninglessly), to be manifest in the present cycle, and to be potential in all future cycles. As Vyāsa puts it in his commentary on I: 28, "When Om repetition and yoga come to perfection, the supreme Self (*paramātman*) shines forth."[24] Or as Śaṅkara elaborates:

> When he [the yogin] is not disturbed by other ideas. . . ., he is perfect in repetition and in yoga; by that perfection in repetition and meditation on the supreme Lord (*parameśvara*) the supreme (*paramātman*) who stands in the highest place (*parameṣṭhin*) shines forth for the yogin.[25]

This result is surely far removed from empty mindlessness that the ritual chanting of *AUM* implied to Heiler and, I suspect, to most modern persons.

Finally, the text then asks, when the yogin has reached the *nirvicāra* state of full realization of Īśvara's perfection, what happens then? From the *nirvicāra* state, says *Yoga Sūtra* I: 29, comes realization of the devotee's own self, and the absence of all obstacles. Vyāsa comments:

> As a result of devotion to the Lord [Īśvara], there are none of the obstacles like illness, and he has a perception of his own true nature. As the Lord is a Puruṣa, pure, radiant, alone and beyond evil, so the Puruṣa in him, witness of the buddhi, knows him to be.[26]

Śaṅkara notes in his gloss that the words "As the Lord is a Puruṣa. . . ., so. . . ." highlight the difference between the *puruṣa* of Īśvara and the devotee's realization of his own *puruṣa*. While the devotee had to free himself from the bondage in *karma-saṁsāra*, Īśvara is different and unique in that he has always been free.[27]

Our careful study of *Yoga Sūtra* I: 24–29 has shown in a most detailed way how the power of scriptural words (*āgama*) as manifested in Īśvara gives not only supersensuous or divine knowledge but also a practical means for the realization of release. According to the Yoga tradition, it was this route of devotion to Īśvara that was chosen by most of yogis as their path to release.[28]

CONCLUSION

In contrast with Nietzsche's view of language as a "prison house" or the modern structuralist view of language as an alien system weighing down human consciousness, the *Yoga Sūtras* of Patañjali with the commentaries of Vyasa, Vachaspati Mishra, and Śaṅkara offer an analysis of language as having inherent within itself the power to convey knowledge (both sensuous and supersensuous) and to realize release. The *Yoga Sūtras* claim that ordinary words which report the perceptions and inferences of a clear mind can convey that knowledge by verbal communication (*āgama*) to another person. *Āgama* in this sense is judged by Yoga to be a *pramāṇa* or source of valid knowledge, along with inference and perception. When it comes to knowledge of the supersensuous or divine, *āgama* can also help us but it must be the *āgama* or word of a special person—a *puruṣa* who was never obscured by karmic obstruction. Īśvara, claims Vyasa's commentary on the *Yoga Sūtras*, is such a special *puruṣa*, and his words are the Vedic scriptures given to the *Ṛśis* at the beginning of each cycle of creation. Through these Vedas, then, we have valid knowledge of the supersensuous which Īśvara has directly "seen." But can these special words of scripture enable us to realize release from *karma-saṁsāra*. "Yes" answers the *Yoga Sūtras*, especially the special word "*AUM*," which as the beginningless utterance of Īśvara is the seed from which the Vedas arise. By meditatively chanting *AUM*, the devotee will gradually purify his or her mind until the highest level of *nirvicāra samādhi* is realized. Then the fully purified perception of Īśvara as the eternally pure *puruṣa* and original speaker of the Vedas opens the door to the devotee's realization of his or her own *puruṣa* as also pure and free.

The *Yoga Sūtra*'s attribution of knowledge and spiritual power to *āgama*, as anchored in the pure *sattva* body of Īśvara, calls into question Eliade's rather flippant remark that when all is said and done Patañjali's introduction of Īśvara into Sāṅkhya soteriology is perfectly useless.[29] In strictly theoretical terms Eliade may be correct in his view that there was already a soteriological impulse in *prakṛti* and therefore no special help from Īśvara on the Vedas is needed. But the fact remains that without Īśvara, *āgama* would give no special knowledge from the Vedas or special help via the chanting of *AUM*. While it would still be theoretically possible to realize self-knowledge, in practice it would be most difficult since the last two *niyamas*, or aids to yoga practice, would have been removed along with all of *Yoga Sūtras* I: 24–29. According to the Yoga tradition *Īśvara-praṇidhāna* (focusing the mind upon *Īśvara*) and *svādhyāya* (in the form of the mantra chanting of *AUM*) has been the core practice of most yogis. Add to that the evidence that it is precisely the Īśvara aspect of Yogic *āgama* that Śaṅkara seems to have Vedāntinized in his Vivaraṇa gloss on Vyāsa's commentary, and it is clear that more attention must be given to Īśvara and *āgama* in the *Yoga Sūtras* than Eliade was prepared to allow.

3

The Yoga Psychology Underlying Bhartṛhari's *Vākyapadīya*

In the previous chapter we saw how the function of language as valid knowledge and the Vedas as divine truth were given psychological explanation by Patañjali in his *Yoga Sūtras*. This chapter turns to the analysis of how words and sentence function according to Bhartṛhari, India's greatest philosopher of language. Living after Patañjali, Bhartṛhari (c. 500 CE) undoubtedly knew the *Yoga Sūtras* and the understanding of language and the Vedas put forth by Patañjali (described in chapter 2). In this chapter we examine how Patañjali's Yoga psychology is assumed by Bhartṛhari in writing his great work, the *Vākyapadīya* (The Philosophy of Word and Sentence).

The seventh-century Chinese pilgrim to India, I-tsing, reports in his diary that in the education curriculum of the day Bhartṛhari's *Vākyapadīya*, or Philosophy of Word and Sentence, was the crowning work studied by the most serious students. Yoga was the traditional psychology of India in Bhartṛhari's day, and indeed has continued to occupy that status in the minds of most Indians right up to the present. It is only during the last few decades that the psychology taught in Indian universities and colleges has come to be modern empirical or scientific psychology. As noted in the introduction, the classic formulation of traditional Yoga psychology is the *Yoga Sūtras* of Patañjali, which are usually dated around 200 CE. The important commentary, or *bhāṣya*, on the *Yoga Sūtras* is attributed to Vyāsa, and seems to be contemporary with Bhartṛhari. Later, an explanation, or ṭīkā, called the *Tattva-Vāicāradī*, written by Vācaspati Miśra, was added. Although the *Yoga Sūtras* are written within the context of the Sāṅkhya school of metaphysics,[1] the focus throughout is on the analysis of the psychological processes commonly accepted by all of the various schools, orthodox and heterodox alike, as described at the beginning of the introduction.

An understanding of this commonly assumed Yoga psychology is necessary if Bhartṛhari's *Vākyapadīya* (and his thought generally) is to be seen in its full perspective. A complete analysis of the *Vākyapadīya* must include both its philosophical aspect (i.e., the metaphysical inquiry into the nature of meaning in language) and its psychological aspect (i.e., the Yoga explanation of the processes required for communicating meaning at the lower level of language, and the discipline for becoming one with the Divine Word, *śabdapūrvayoga*). In current writing on the *Vākyapadīya*, scholars such as K. A. S. Iyer[2] and G. Sastri[3] have concentrated on the first aspect, the metaphysics, and largely neglected the second, the psychological and practical aspects.[4] In this study a conscious effort is made to give equal treatment to both aspects. In this chapter an attempt is made at describing the Yoga psychology assumed by Bhartṛhari but often left unstated. Not only will this provide a more complete picture of Bhartṛhari's theory of language; it will also suggest in detail what he may have meant by *śabdapūrvayoga* as a discipline for meditation upon the Divine Word until *mokṣa*, or union with Śabdabrahman (Divine Word-Consciousness) is realized.[5]

THE STRUCTURE OF CONSCIOUSNESS AS ŚABDABRAHMAN

Vākyapadīya I: 123 describes consciousness as an intertwined unity of cognition and word that constantly seeks to manifest itself in speech. A conception of consciousness that seems parallel to Bhartṛhari's description is found in the *Yoga Sūtra* analysis of Īśvara's omniscience which we examined in the previous chapter.[6] Here the intertwining of word and meaning in consciousness is seen in its purest form. Within Īśvara's consciousness is the seed form of all words, which remains constant throughout the various manifestations and dissolutions of each cycle of creation. Every new cycle arises out of the need of Īśvara's consciousness to burst forth into expression. Thus Īśvara, or the Lord, is described as having two characteristics: a pure consciousness of perfect quality (*sattva*) and as being the germ or seed (*bija*) of omniscience at its utmost excellence.[7]

Let us briefly review the detailed description of this special consciousness of Īśvara undertaken in Yoga psychology through an analysis of one's own experience of consciousness. In one's ordinary experience of consciousness, three aspects or substantive qualities (*guṇas*) are found: *sattva*, which is brightness or intelligence; *rajas*, which is passion or energy; and *tamas*, which is dullness or inertia. Although each of these *guṇas* keeps its own separate identity, no individual *guṇa* ever exists independently. Rather, the three *guṇas* are always necessarily found together like three strands of a rope. However, the proportionate composition of consciousness assigned to each of the *guṇas* is constantly changing.[8] Only the predominant *guṇa* will be easily recognized in a particular thought. The other two *guṇas* will be present but subordinate, and therefore their presence will have to be determined by inference.

In the case of Īśvara, as we saw in chapter 2, his consciousness is described as being completely dominated by pure *sattva*. Within this *sattva* there is a teleology that ensures the reappearance of Īśvara in each new creation for the purpose of communicating to all beings his omniscient knowledge, so that they may, with the help of his grace, attain *mokṣa*. The psychological mechanism by which Īśvara's reappearance in each new creation is ensured is as follows. At the end of each creation, Īśvara freely wishes that his *sattva* consciousness should appear again at the time of the next creation. This wish leaves behind a *saṁskāra*, or mental potency, which acts as a "seed state" from which Īśvara blossoms afresh in each new creation. The underlying metaphysical assumption here (from Bhartṛhari's perspective) is that Brahman freely phenomenalizes himself as Īśvara as an act of grace so as to provide the means (i.e., the revelation of the Veda) by which one can attain *mokṣa*. On the psychological level, this revelation, if it is to be capable of human understanding, must function through human cognition. Thus there is a kind of continuum between Īśvara's *sattva* and that of the lowest being (*jīva*).

The matchless perfection of Īśvara's *sattva* consciousness is evident in, and attested to by, his omniscience, which he communicates to the *ṛśis* as scriptural truth, or *āgama* (including *śruti*, *smṛti*, the epics, and the Purāṇas). The psychological means by which this communication takes place is technically referred to as *viśiṣṭopahita* (intuition caused by the grace of a special person). The *ṛṣi* supersensuously sees directly into the omniscience incarnated in Īśvara's *sattva* and reveals it to other persons in the manifested form of uttered speech—Veda, the authoritative *vāk*. Īśvara is thus named both the first knower and the first teacher, who, out of grace, gives to the great *ṛṣis* a direct vision of that which is the essence of all language and all revelation, namely, his own consciousness. Within each creation, at least, this unity of omniscience and consciousness, which is Īśvara's *sattva*, is timeless in that it continues on unchanging, although the limitations necessary for human language are constantly being placed upon it.[9] It is the dynamic ground upon which all language and knowledge rests and from which all speech evolves. Scriptural truth, both as the revealed word (*śruti*) and the remembered writings of tradition (*smṛti*), is really the authoritative verbalization of Īśvara's *sattva*, and may therefore be taken as the expression of the true nature of consciousness.[10] All this is expressed in the one mystic symbol, *AUM*, which, when spoken, connotes Īśvara with all his power for omniscience.

Īśvara, as described above, represents for Yoga psychology the pure ideal upon which the Yogin, or devotee, should focus in his daily practice. As noted in chapter 2, Īśvara is defined as a special kind of being who is free from or untouched by what we might call instinctual drives (*kleśas*) and the actions or thoughts performed as a result of such drives (*karma*).[11] When all these aspects of psychological functioning are deleted, what is left is Īśvara's omniscient consciousness with its compassionate telos for communication. It is in this sense that Īśvara is a close parallel to Bhartṛhari's *Vākyapadīya* conception of consciousness as a given unity of thought and meaning. The Yoga conception of Īśvara provides, as required by the *Vākyapadīya*, that consciousness contain within it the seed state of omniscience. And just as the *Yoga Sūtras* take this omniscient consciousness as the universal basis for the scriptural truth (*āgama*) of the *ṛṣis*, so also Bhartṛhari conceives of *āgama* as necessarily existing within all beings and providing the basis for their *pratibhā*, or divine consciousness, experience. Although there may be some differences in Bhartṛhari's concept of *āgama*, the main outline of his conception is in agreement with that of Patañjali.[12] For Bhartṛhari in the very first verse of the *Vākyapadīya*, Brahman is conceived of as the omniscient word-principle, the *Śabdatattva*. Bhartṛhari maintains that the Veda is not only the means of attaining *mokṣa*, but is also the image (*anukāra*) of Brahman. This is almost identical to the *Yoga Sūtra* description of Īśvara as the ever free and eternal Lord whose omniscience, verbalized as Veda, enables beings to achieve *mokṣa*.

While all this indicates good grounds for the use of Patañjali's psychological analysis of Īśvara as a parallel against which to interpret Bhartṛhari's conception of reality as word-consciousness or *Śabdabrahman*, one difference does exist at the level of the highest metaphysical speculation. The Yoga system is ultimately a duality between pure consciousness (*puruṣa*) and nonintelligent matter (*prakṛti*). Consequently, Vācaspati points out that Īśvara's *sattva* does not possess the power of consciousness, since *sattva* is nonintelligent in its own nature.[13] From the viewpoint of Sāṅkhya-Yoga metaphysics, *sattva*, as a manifestation of *prakṛti*, only appears to have intelligence as a result of *avidyā* or the beginningless wrong identification between *puruṣa* and *prakṛti*.[14] The nature of *prakṛti* is also exemplified in terms of causation, namely, that the cause persists in all its effects, and therefore the nature of the cause can be deduced by observing what persists in the effects. For example, gold may be seen to exist in all objects made from gold. By looking at them, it can be inferred that gold is the original material out of which they were all made.

Although Bhartṛhari's *sphoṭa* theory of language is nondualistic, there is evidence of a similar sort of causal argument. In the *vṛtti*, or commentary on the *Vākyapadīya* 1: 123, it is stated that our knowledge of everything in the world is interwoven with the word. Knowledge is by its nature in the form of words. In order to cognize any object, we must first cognize the word relating to it. Therefore, since all manifestations of Brahman are intertwined with the word, so also the root cause of all such manifestations, Brahman, must be of the nature of the word (*Śabdatattva*). From Bhartṛhari's viewpoint, therefore, Īśvara's omniscient *sattva*, as the root cause of all speech, needs no outside illumination (such as *puruṣa*), for as the ultimate Word-Principle (*Śabdatattva*), it is self-luminous. Now, from the Yoga standpoint, for the practical purpose of our psychological experience, Īśvara's *sattva* also appears to us as self-illuminated in nature. It is only at the level of *mokṣa*, or final discrimination, leading directly to *kaivalya* (realization of the *puruṣa's* existence as a self independent and free from the fetters of *prakṛti*) that the Sāṅkhya-Yoga dualistic metaphysics results in a total break with Bhartṛhari's theory. At the empirical level of verbal communication between individuals, however, there is no difficulty, since for psychological purposes both Yoga and *sphoṭa* treat consciousness as being self-manifesting.[15]

The above discussion shows that in the Yoga conception of Īśvara there is a readymade basis for a psychological interpretation of the *Vākyapadīya* view of consciousness. In that discussion, the psychological mechanism by which the noumenal word forms of Īśvara or the *Śabdatattva* exist from one cycle of creation to the next was identified as *saṁskāra*. *Saṁskāra* is defined as follows. When a particular mental state (*citta vṛtti*) passes away into another, it does not totally disappear but is preserved within consciousness as a latent form or *saṁskāra*.[16] Such *saṁskāra's* are always tending to manifest themselves anew, and therefore are also referred to as *bīja*, or seed states. Īśvara's state of *sattvic* omniscience is described as *bīja* in that his matured omniscience lays down the seeds for its own eternal continuance both within and between creations. The "seed" connotation emphasizes potency, which is the essential characteristic of *saṁskāra*. On the analogy of the seed and the sprout, *saṁskāras* are seen to be self-perpetuating in nature. A particular mental state, or *citta vṛtti*, results in a like *saṁskāra*, which is always attempting to manifest itself in another mental state similar to the first.

Thus, there is a self-generating cycle from mental state to *saṁskāras* to mental state, and so on. In Yoga thinking this cycle is beginningless (i.e., it has always been going on) but not necessarily endless. Although the repetition of the same series of mental state-*saṁskāra*-mental state results in the establishing and strengthening of habit patterns (*vāsanās*), which are likened to "roots" that have grown deep within the "soil" of consciousness, the continual practicing of an opposing *saṁskāra* series will eventually weaken and render the "root," or *vāsanā*, of the less-reinforced series impotent.

In Yoga thought such *saṁskāra* series or *vāsanās* are categorized as either (1) *kliṣṭa* (afflicted by ignorance), obstructing and leading away from the revelation of knowledge or insight (*prajñā*); or (2) *akliṣṭa* (unafflicted), leading toward *prajñā*.[17] Seen in this perspective, *citta*, or consciousness, is like a constantly moving river whose flow can go in either of two directions—or both ways at the same time.[18] Through the *saṁskāra* series resulting from Īśvara's beginningless bestowing of the Veda within consciousness, the mind has an inherent tendency toward knowledge and the revelation of Brahman. But through the *kliṣṭa-saṁskāra* series composed of beginningless ignorance (*avidyā*) and egoity (*asmitā*), which characterize the endless round of birth-death-rebirth, the mind has an innate tendency toward ignorance.[19] The teleology of consciousness (via the grace of Īśvara), however, ensures that the will to realize knowledge is never lost; thus the innate overall tendency of consciousness is to flow in the direction of knowledge.

How does this Yoga analysis of consciousness and its *saṁskāra* function apply to the *Vākyapadīya*? Bhartṛhari's *sphoṭa* theory defines consciousness as an intertwined unity of cognition and word which constantly seeks to manifest itself in speech. In the Yoga analysis of consciousness, we have seen how the *sattva* aspect of *citta* is beginninglessly endowed with the word forms or meanings of the Veda because of the grace of Īśvara. These *sattvic* word forms are equivalent to Bhartṛhari's *vākya-sphoṭas*, or sentence meanings. *Saṁskāra* series provide the psychological process by which the *sphoṭas* become and continue as *vṛttis*, or states within consciousness. Such a primordial noumenal *sphoṭa* is psychologically analyzed as a concentrated insight (*prajñā*) that exists as an undisturbed succession of pure *akliṣṭa saṁskāra*. It does not fluctuate or change, nor does it require any supporting object (*ālambana*), since it is itself the substratum—the eternal universal essence upon which all phenomenal language manifestations of that word depend.[20] As *prajñā*, or pure intuition, it is unitary, partless, and free from the predicate relations that characterize ordinary speech. Yet as consciousness, it contains in addition to this pure *sattvic* intuition elements of *tamas* and *rajas* (especially the latter), which provide the material and motive force for the phenomenalization of the *sphoṭa* into thought and speech. Thus, the inherent telos of consciousness is toward the self-revelation and communication of which Bhartṛhari speaks.

The actual processes of phenomenalization have not as yet been analyzed. Up to this point, the focus has been on the analysis of consciousness at the noumenal or *paśyantī* level in order to demonstrate its nature as including cognition, word-meaning, and the desire for speech. The mention of phenomenalization here is simply to indicate that the *rajas* and *tamas* aspects of consciousness provide the potential for its various particular manifestations.

PSYCHOLOGICAL PROCESSES IN SPEAKING

In the above-mentioned examination of the nature of consciousness, a description has been offered of how consciousness could contain within itself (in a potential state) word, cognition, and the desire for expression. This level of consciousness has been shown to be synonymous with *paśyantī vāk* or *Śabdabrahman* in the *Vākyapadīya*. Here the *sphoṭa* exists in an undifferentiated state. It is simply the *vāk* (word) of Īśvara pervasively existing within undifferentiated consciousness in eternally continuous pure *sattva saṁskāra* series. In it there is no distinction between word and meaning, but only the constant presence of meaning as a whole. There is present, however, "a going out," a desire for expression. It is this characteristic of consciousness that will be focused on now.

An introspective examination of one's initial experience in the act of speaking provides the starting point. At its earliest genesis the speaking act would seem to involve the following: some kind of mental effort to control or tune out distracting sensations and thoughts, an inwardly focused concentration of the mind, and an effort of the mind to bring into self-awareness some idea (or glimpse of reality) that is only vaguely within our ken. Although we may feel very sure of its presence just beyond the fringes of our conscious awareness, and although we may find ourselves impelled by a great desire to reveal that idea in discursive thought, a strong effort at concentrated thinking is often required before any clear conception of it is mentally achieved. Even then one may well feel dissatisfied in that the laboriously conceived conceptualization proves to be so inadequate and incomplete in comparison with one's direct intuition of the noumenal "idea" that remains stubbornly transcendent in the face of all one's attempts to capture it in discrete thought. Yet the more persistently and intensely one thinks, the clearer one's corresponding intuition of the object often becomes. But thinking it is not enough. One is also conscious of a compulsion to manifest one's inner thought in speech (or writing), for only then does the urge for the revelation of the hidden idea seem fully satisfied. According to Bhartṛhari, it is this urge or inner energy (*kratu*) that is responsible for the whole process of the manifestation of consciousness and the expression of *sphoṭa* or meaning-whole in both inner thought and outer speech.[21]

Bhartṛhari maintains that this *kratu*, or inner energy, is a quality of the *sphoṭa* itself. But the telos of *kratu* to burst forth (*sphuṭ*) into disclosure is experienced within self-awareness in two forms. On the one hand, there is the pent-up energy for disclosure residing in the *sphoṭa*, while on the other hand there is the epistemic urge of the subjective consciousness and its desire, as a speaker, to communicate.[22] According to Yoga, what would be the psychological processes involved in speaking forth the *sphoṭa* (idea or meaning-whole)?

In Yoga theory it is clear that the energy aspect of any manifestation of consciousness will be directly attributable to *rajas*. We have already described consciousness in its unmanifested state (*paśyantī vāk*) as containing the omniscience bestowed by Īśvara's *sattva*. The characteristic of this state is that in it *sattva* predominates over *rajas* and *tamas* in a steady flow of Īśvara's omniscient ideas (Vedas). These ideas, or unmanifested *sphoṭas*, are but limitations within *sattva* of the pure universal knowledge of consciousness. At this level of collective consciousness (*buddhitattva*), there is no subject-object distinction, and, as Vyāsa puts it, "all we can say is that it exists."[23] This *buddhitattva* is consciousness in its most universal form, containing within it all the *buddhis,* or intellects, of individuals and potentially all the matter of which the gross world is formed. Thus it is also referred to as *mahat,* or "the great one," in Yoga writings.

Now, as a result of the teleology inherent in consciousness (i.e., the grace of Īśvara), the *buddhitattva* is affected by its own pent-up *rajas* activity, which posits itself as ego (*ahaṁkāra*). This is the sense of "I-ness," "me," or "mine." Due to the increasing preponderance of *rajas guṇa* in the originally pure *sattva* of *buddhi,* the *buddhi* consciousness transforms itself into the ego, the subject or the knower. But at this first phase of ego manifestation the ego, although conscious of itself, has as yet no other content to know since the *tamas guṇa* is still under suppression. This bare "I-ness" is a preponderance of *rajas* as manifested by *sattva,* which knows itself to be active and holds itself as the permanent energizing activity of all the phenomena of life.[24] Still, however, there is no subject-object distinction and therefore the *sphoṭas* inherent in consciousness can only be known as a general datum of consciousness but with the characteristic of "I-ness" or "mine." *Sphoṭa* at this level is described as the subtle inner word (*sūkṣmā vāk*) that becomes the knower (*jñātā*), and then in order to reveal itself becomes the external word.[25] In the Yoga description the *ahaṁkāra,* or ego, is equivalent to the *sūkṣmā vāk,* and *rajas* to the *sakti,* or power of *vāk* for self-manifestation.

The next level of manifestation occurs when the *buddhi* consciousness, through the *ahaṁkāra,* turns back upon itself and divides into a part that sees and a part that is seen—the subject-object distinction that characterizes thought. According to Yoga theory, consciousness accomplishes this involutional bifurcation by virtue of the germs of subjectivity and objectivity that the *guṇas* of consciousness contain within themselves. At the initial *ahaṁkāra* level, these two sides of subject and object exist, but only in an implicit way within the bare self-awareness. This bifurcated individuation of the *buddhi* through the *ahaṁkāra* occurs by the instrumental activity of *rajas* in evolving, on the one hand, a *sattva* preponderance and, on the other, a *tamas* preponderance of consciousness.

Following first the *rajas*-produced *sattva* preponderance, it is seen as a continuing individuation of the *buddhitattva,* or collective consciousness, since the latter was already characterized as having a dominance of *sattva.* By the further activity of *rajas,* the *sattva* consciousness through the *ahaṁkāra* develops itself into the five cognitive senses (*jñanendriya*) of vision, touch, smell, taste, and hearing; the five action faculties (*karmendriya*) of speaking, handling, locomotion, evacuation, and sexual generation; and the *prāṇas,* or *vayus* (psychomotor activities) that help both action and cognition and are the life-force manifestations of *rajas.* Also formed by the *rajas* activity in the *sattva* preponderance is a further specialization of the *ahaṁkāra* as *manas* (mind), the instrument whereby the *ahaṁkāra* directly connects itself with the cognitive and conative senses. It is in this manner that Yoga theory envisages the collective consciousness of the *buddhitattva* being individuated into the intellects (individual *buddhis*) of finite persons. Dasgupta helpfully summarizes this *rajas*-produced individuation of citta:

> The individual ahaṁkāras and senses are related to the individual buddhis by his developing sattva determinations from which they had come into being. Each buddhi with its own group of ahaṁkāra (ego) and sense-evolutes thus forms a microcosm separate from similar other buddhis with their associated groups. So far therefore as knowledge is subject to sense-influence and the ego, it is different for each individual, but so far as a general mind (*kāraṇa buddhi*) apart from sense knowledge is concerned, there is a community of all buddhis in the buddhitattva. Even there, however, each buddhi is separated from other buddhis by its own peculiarly associated ignorance (*avidyā*).[26]

From the viewpoint of the *Vākyapadīya*, the above situation is interpreted as follows. At the collective level each *buddhi* has incorporated in its particular *avidyā vāsanās* accumulated from word usage in previous lives. These are seed forms of the inherent *śabda* (word) vocalization patterns, which, as Bhartṛhari points out, are seen to already exist in the newborn baby who does not yet know any language. This is the expressive element of *sphoṭa* in its potential state. But insofar as the individual *buddhi* participates in the general mind (the *buddhitattva*), the *sattva* there encountered contains seed forms of the inherent meanings, described above as Vedic *akliṣṭa saṁskāra* series bestowed by the grace of Īśvara. These seeds are the meaning elements (*artha*) in potential form, and are also referred to as the expressed aspect of the *sphoṭa*.

On the other side of the bifurcation by the activity of *rajas*, the *tamas guṇa* of the *buddhitattva* individuates through the *ahaṁkāra* into the five *tanmātras*, or subtle elements, which, by a further evolution of themselves, produce the five gross elements of matter. The *tamas guṇa* by itself is inert mass, but in combination with *rajas* becomes fully dynamic and vibrant, in somewhat the same sense as matter is conceived as moving electrical energy charges in modern physics and chemistry. In its state as mere mass, *tamas* is referred to as *bhūtādi*. By its combination with differing amounts of energy (*rajas*), the *bhūtādi* is individuated into various *tanmātras*, or aggregations of the original mass-units. Due to their particular collocations of mass and energy, the *tanmātras* possess the potential physical qualities of sound (*śabda*), touch (*sparśa*), color or shape (*rūpa*), flavor or taste (*rasa*), and smell (*gandha*). These *tanmātras* are the subtle material counterparts of the five cognitive senses that formed part of the *rajas-sattva* individuation described above.

Consciousness, or *citta*, having reached the furthest limit of its *rajas* individuation by producing the senses and *manas* on the one side and the material atoms on the other, should not be thought of as having reached the end of its process of change. The underlying principle of *citta's* transformation is concisely stated by Dasgupta: "The order of succession is not from whole to parts nor from parts to whole but ever from a relatively less differentiated, less determinate, less coherent whole to a relatively more determinate, more coherent whole. . . . Increasing differentiation proceeds *pari passu* with increasing integration within the evolving whole."[27] Seen in its cosmic perspective, the *rajas*-energized transformation of *sattva* and *tamas* toward both individuation and integration results in a totality of mass, energy, and illumination that remains constant throughout its diversity of collocations. Although manifestations of the *guṇas* within individual *buddhis* may appear to be subject to growth and decay, the *guṇas*, taken in the totality of their manifested and unmanifested *citta*, are a cosmic constant with no overall increase or decrease but having a continuous circular flow within the system as a whole.

In Yoga theory it seems clear that *rajas* activity provides the psychological basis required for the "instinctive urge" to phenomenalize the *sphoṭa*. *Rajas*, in its pent-up state within the *buddhitattva*, is a clear description of the energy for disclosure (*sphuṭ*) that Bhartṛhari conceives of as residing within the *sphoṭa*. And in its individuation of the *buddhitattva* through the *ahaṁkāra*, *rajas* has demonstrated its power to produce the subject-object distinction that characterizes speech at its two lower levels. The formation of the *ahaṁkāra*, with its sense of egoity, provides for the overall sense of awareness, which, in its more individuated forms as mind and senses, forms the basis for the experiencing of epistemic curiosity. At the finite level of ego, mind, and senses, such an epistemic drive has been shown to provide both the desire to bring into self-awareness Bhartṛhari's hidden meaning (*artha*) of *sphoṭa* and the subsequent urge to express that revelation in uttered speech (*dhvani*). Now that the instinctive or dynamic basis for expression of *sphoṭa* has been described, the speaking act itself and its fully individuated manifestation of the *sphoṭa* as word-meaning (*artha*) and word-sound (*dhvani*) will be examined.

In Yoga psychology, perception may be thought of as being either external or internal. External perception, of course, occurs through the sense organs. Internal perception is said to occur via the internal mental organ (*antaḥkaraṇa*), which assumes the threefold character of *buddhi*, *ahaṁkāra*, and *manas* accordingly as its functions differ. The *buddhi* functions as the discriminating, knowing intellect, the *ahaṁkāra* as providing perception with the ego-sense of "mine," and the *manas* as the processing or liaison center between perceptive and motor activity. It should be noted here that in Yoga theory, names such as *buddhi*, *ahaṁkāra*, and *manas* are used, not to refer to any kind of structural division within consciousness, but rather as an attempt to functionally describe the unified functioning of the whole *antaḥkaraṇa*, or mind.

In its *buddhi* function, the *antaḥkaraṇa* contains the *saṁskāras* or memory traces of both the word-meanings (*arthas*) and the word-sounds (*dhvanis*—vocalization patterns from previous lives). In its *ahaṁkāra* function, the *antaḥkaraṇa* has the first awareness of the universal *artha*, or meaning, as its own cognition, and the concomitant awareness of the forming of that *artha* into inner speech, or *dhvani*. In the introspection of one's speaking act, this represents the cognitive birth of the earliest formulations in one's grasping of the whole idea, or *vākya sphoṭa*. The initial distinctions between *artha* and *dhvani* are therefore manifesting themselves.

At this stage, the *manas* aspect of the *antaḥkaraṇa* is coordinating the concomitant developing vocalization patterns into internal thoughts in which the order of words is present. The *dhvani*-thoughts concomitant to the *artha* of the *sphoṭa* in question are psychologically composed by the interaction of the vibrant and highly charged *śabda tanmātra* with the organ of speech. The individuation of the *śabda tanmātra* into a particular *sphoṭa dhvani* manifestation occurs through the conjoint action of a variety of factors. The overall form of the *dhvani* is provided by the *artha* through its "magnetlike" attracting of the *tanmātra* into its (the *arthas*) collateral *dhvani* pattern. But in order for the *śabda tanmātra* to be so structured, the speech organ acts as a variable filter through which the *tanmātra* is limited.[28] It is in this way that *vāsanās* of vocalization patterns from previous lives[29] instrumentally operate through the speech organ so that the speech organ and the electric vibrancy of the *śabda tanmātra* can together respond to the electromagnet-like pattern of the *artha* to produce the *dhvani*. Throughout all of this, the *manas* is providing the psychomotor coordination for the complex cognitive activity involved.

The above-mentioned interpretation provides a practical psychological explanation, in terms of Yoga theory, of how the *sphoṭa* inherently present within the *buddhi* can express itself as *artha* and *dhvani* within individuated consciousness. In the analysis this far, however, *dhvani* is still at the level of thought or inner speech, corresponding to Bhartṛhari's *madhyamā vāk*. In addition to the organ of speech, the *prāṇa*, or breath, will also be involved; the psychomotor activities, such as action of the muscles of the diaphragm, drive the *śabda tanmātra*, in its gross sound form, through the speech organ. In Yoga theory the individuating process is a continuum, so that even at the level of internal thought, the initial gross manifestations of *dhvani* will be present in a subtle fashion. Therefore to move to the final level of individuation requires only that the gross forms, already minutely present, receive further development. Speaking aloud requires only that the processes of one's thought-out sentences be given an increase of *prāṇa*, or breath, until the gross, or *nāda*, articulation of the phonemes occurs.[30] In the case of written speech, a slightly different pattern of the *prāṇa*, or psychomotor structuring, so as to include hand-eye coordination and a learned system of phonetic representation, is all that is required. This is Bhartṛhari's *vaikharī vāk* level of expression, in which what is meant (*artha*) is produced as word-sound (*dhvani*) by the articulatory organs. Thus, interpreted according to Yoga psychology, the *Vākyapadīya* is seen to provide a logical and experienceable explanation of the speaking act.

PSYCHOLOGICAL PROCESSES IN HEARING

In the previous section, the speaking act was described, showing how, according to Yoga psychology, the magnet-like action of the *artha* structured or limited the pervasive *śabda tanmātra* by filtering it through the inherent vocalization patterns (from *vāsanās* of word use in previous lives) of the speech organ so as to produce a *dhvani* or sound continuum, ranging from the subtle speech of inner thought to the gross articulation of the phonemes. Once articulated as configurations of gross atoms patterned by the psychomotor activities of the breath (*prāṇa*), the phonemes continue to vibrate outward in expanding concentric circles from the speaker. The hearing act is initiated when the uttered phonemes in their concentric expansion as configurations of gross atoms, like waves moving outward when a stone is dropped into the water, strike against the hearing organ of the listener. Communication occurs, according to Bhartṛhari, when these sounds striking against the ear as uttered phonemes evoke in the mind of the listener a perception of the same *sphoṭa* from which the speaker began his or her utterance.

But exactly how do these discrete phoneme patterns striking against the ear psychologically function so as to evoke the partless *sphoṭa* inherently residing in each individual *buddhi*? On this question all Bhartṛhari offers are a few suggestions with regard to the function of *saṁskāras* and the general idea that the heard phonemes cognize the *sphoṭa* through a series of perceptions distorted by error; the *sphoṭa* perception following the hearing of the first phoneme has the highest error, and the *sphoṭa* perception following the hearing of the last phoneme has the lowest error. Perhaps the most detailed psychological description of the process occurs in the *vṛtti*. "The sounds [phonemes], while they manifest the word [*sphoṭa*], leave impression-seeds [*saṁskāras*] progressively clearer and conducive to the clear perception (of the word). Then, the final sound brings to the mind which has now attained maturity or a certain fitness by the awakening of the impressions of previous cognitions, the form of the word as coloured by itself."[31] But this is still a rather general analysis. Perhaps a more systematic interpretation can be obtained from Yoga psychology.

Fortunately, *Yoga Sūtra* 111: 17 deals with this exact question. The *sūtra* is stated in terms that seem to provide a very close parallel to those of the *sphoṭa* theory: "*śabda*" is used in the sense of the word-sound, or *dhvani*; "*artha*" is interpreted, as in *sphoṭa* theory, to be the meaning or object; and "*pratyaya*," as the *ālambana* or support for the *śabda* and *artha*, would seem to be very close to the *sphoṭa* of Bhartṛhari. In his *bhāṣya*, Vyāsa analyzes the hearing problem in terms almost identical to those of the *Vākyapadīya*.

> . . . voice has its function [in uttering] only the [sounds of] syllables. And the organ-of-hearing has as its object only that [emission of air] which has been mutated into a sound [by contact with the eight places of articulation belonging to the vocal organ]. But it is a mental-process (*buddhi*) that grasps the word [as significant sound] by seizing the letter-sounds each in turn and binding them together [into one word]. Sounds-of-syllables (*varṇa*) do not naturally aid each other, for they cannot coexist at the same time. Not having attained-to-the-unity-of a word and not having [conveyed a definite meaning], they become audible (*āvis*) and they become inaudible (*tiras*). Hence it is said that individually [letter-sounds] lack the nature of a word.[32]

Vyāsa thus ends up with the same problem as Bhartṛhari, namely, by what psychological mechanism do the ephemeral phonemes heard by the ear become bound together by the *buddhi* into a unity (*sphoṭa*) that manifests the meaning-whole?

Vyāsa begins the discussion of his solution to the problem by suggesting that each phoneme taken by itself is capable of standing for any meaning; it has universal application. But when a letter appears in combination with other letters, the preceding and following letters have the function of restricting or limiting the application of each letter to a particular meaning. Thus there are many uttered sounds, which by being placed in particular orders result in slightly different overall sounds, as determined by convention, and therefore are able to denote a certain meaning (*artha*). For example, the literal sounds of *g*, *au*, and *ḥ*, possessed as they are of the potentiality of giving names to all objects (*arthas*), denote in this particular order (*gauḥ*, "cow") the object that is possessed of udder, dewlap, and so on. Vācaspati adds the comment that a specific sonorous impression is thus established in the *antaḥkaraṇa* as the hearing of the ordered utterance ceases. The specific sonorous impression that is evoked in the mind is the single image of the word *gauḥ*. This mental unity, or *sphoṭa*, which is commonly called a word, has no parts or sequence within itself and reveals a meaning-object that is also one. The sequence of the uttered phonemes, as the last one is heard by the ear, reveals the one mental image of the *sphoṭa*. But what exactly is the psychological process by which this inner revelation of the one by the many heard phonemes takes place?

The solution offered by Vyāsa and Vācaspati is actually the logical counterpart of the process described in the last section, by which the *artha* of a particular *sphoṭa* resulted in the utterance of its particular vocalization of *śabda tanmātra* through the speech organ. The distinctive pattern of *dhvani* produced by the speech organ was described as being the resultant of the *saṁskāras* of speech patterns from previous lives and the "magnet-like" attraction of the *artha*. In the case of hearing, the particular phoneme sequence of the utterance approaches the ear as airwave modulations. The ear, because of its *sattvic*-dominated composition, responds to the magnet-like sound-wave pattern that was originally induced by the action of the *artha* on the *śabda tanmātra*. The *sattvic* aspect of the hearing organ thus begins with the hearing of the first phoneme to approximate (vibrate in tune with) the total sound pattern sent out by the speaker. This sympathetic "vibration," which then travels throughout the consciousness of the hearer, induces maturation of the same *sphoṭa saṁskāra* series in the *buddhi* of the listener.[33] As the subsequent phonemes of the whole spoken pattern strike upon the ear, the sympathetic vibration induced within the hearer's *buddhi* more and more closely approximates the total sound pattern of the gross sound. With the hearing of the last phoneme, its particular "vibration" taken together with the "vibrations" of the preceding phonemes—still active within the *buddhi* by virtue of their self-induced *saṁskāras*—triggers a recognition of the inherent *sphoṭa* in the listener's buddhi.[34]

In this way a complete circle is established from speaker's *sphoṭa* to uttered phonemes to heard phonemes to perception of same *sphoṭa* within hearer. But if there is a completely closed circle from speaker's *sphoṭa* to hearer's *sphoṭa*, including both the *sattva*-dominated levels of the *buddhi* and the grosser levels of the external organs, and if consciousness has an inherent telos toward full revelation of the *sphoṭa* (as Īśvara's omniscience), then why is it that in our speech experience meaning seems to be conveyed in a mediate and often unclear fashion by the series of heard phonemes, rather than in a perfectly clear, immediate fashion by the unitary *sphoṭa*?

The reason for this obscuring of the circle of speech was previously seen, in the speaking act, to be due both to the finite nature of the individuated *manas* and speech organ, necessitating the expression of the noumenal whole in phenomenal parts, and to the obscuring of the meaning by the beginningless *avidyā*. The *avidyā*, or ignorance, referred to is the taking of the uttered letters and words produced by the organ of speech, *manas*, *prāṇa*, et cetera, to be the ultimate word. For these reasons the *sphoṭa* when spoken as a series of phonemes or sound vibrations is already considerably obscured and divided on its arrival at the hearer's ear. The hearer, through his or her own individuated consciousness, then has the task of trying to get back to the partless intuition of the *sphoṭa* from which the speaker began. The fact that the original *sphoṭa*, due to its pervasive existence in the *buddhitattva*, is already potentially present throughout the hearer's *buddhi sattva* and its individuations into *ahaṁkāra*, *manas*, and organ of hearing, paves the way for its recognition. As was the case in the speaking act, *saṁskāras* from our language-use in previous lives pervade the *manas* and the hearing organ so that the natural correlation between a sound pattern of uttered phonemes and its intended *artha* has become intensified through usage in accordance with the consensus of the elders or *saṅketa*.[35]

Although this *saṅketa* intensification of the natural correlation has the positive function of helping the hearer to perceive the *sphoṭa* intended by the speaker, it has at the same time an obscuring (*avidyā*) effect described by both Bhartṛhari and Vyāsa as *adhyāsa*, or superimposition. Bhartṛhari says that the conventional understanding of the uttered words as being one with the meaning is a case of *adhyāsa*.[36] The meaning whole is superimposed upon the parts, but the obscuring *avidya* of *vaikharī* speech is such that the true direction of the superimposition is not realized, and the *ālambana* or ground of the hearing is taken to be the gross sound pattern rather than the *sphoṭa*. Vyāsa says that our taking of the uttered and heard phoneme word pattern to be something real in itself is a result of common understanding (*sampratipatti*). "It is owing to our knowing what this [word] means in accordance with conventional-usage that we attempt to divide it [into sounds of syllables]."[37] Vācaspati shows that psychologically the expression of the word is really a single *vṛtti*, or effort of articulation, as is evidenced by the particular order and unity that makes the utterance of r-a-s-a completely distinct from the word s-a-r-a. The listener also distinguishes between these two words in that the hearing of each word-whole is also done by a functional whole, or single consciousness state, in spite of the fact that conventional usage and grammatical analysis seem to suggest a series of single states, one for each letter.[38] Vyāsa explains psychologically the conventional error as a result of the mutual superimposition or mixing up in the mind of the uttered sounds (*śabda*), the meaning (*artha*), and the *ālambana pratyaya* (*sphoṭa*).

Before describing the detailed analysis of this mixed-up state of *vaikharī* hearing, brief note will be taken of the way in which Yoga psychology, in agreement with the *Vākyapadīya*, interprets the single consciousness state evoked in the hearing of the word as being ultimately the sentence *sphoṭa* rather than word *sphoṭa*. In all perceived words, says Vyāsa, there is the inherent hearing of the *vākya-sphoṭa*, or unitary sentence meaning. If the word *tree* is uttered, the single hearing effort inherently includes within it the verb *is* (*asti*), since no intended meaning (*artha*) can lack existence. Thus the single consciousness state within the listener is the *vākya sphoṭa* "It is a tree." Similarly in the case of the utterance of a single word that is a verb (e.g., *cooks*), the single hearing effort of the listener perceives the agent and any other expansions required as being present in *vākya sphoṭa* (e.g., "Chaitra cooks rice in the vessel on the fire").[39] In *Yoga Sūtra* 111: 17, with its commentaries, we have therefore found a faithful psychological interpretation of Bhartṛhari's thesis that the sentence-meaning is the indivisible unit of speech (*vākya-sphoṭa*), and that ultimately it is the only real (*satya*).[40] The above Yoga interpretation of the hearing event has also outlined the very mixing together of *dhvani*, *artha*, and *sphoṭa* that Bhartṛhari has defined as *vāk* at the *vaikharī*, or gross, level.

In *Yoga Sūtra* 1: 42 we find an even more detailed psychological analysis of *vaikharī vāk*. Here the same technical terms *śabda* and *artha* are used (corresponding to the *sphoṭa* "*dhvani*" and "*artha*"), but instead of *pratyaya* the word *jñāna* is employed to refer to the idea, or sphoṭa. These three are described by Patañjali as being mixed up or superimposed on one another in various predicate relations (*vikalpas*) so that the intended meaning of the word is not clearly seen. In line with *sphoṭa* theory, Vācaspati notes that these predicate relations among *śabda*, *artha*, and *jñāna* represent the diversity that there is in one thing and the identity that there is in diverse things. For example, in *vaikharī* speech, a hearer of the sound pattern "cow" finds, on Yogic introspection, that three possibilities present themselves: (1) there is a predicate relation in which the *śabda* and *jñāna* are dominated and appropriated by the artha "cow"; (2) there is a predicate relation in which *jñāna* and *artha* are dominated and appropriated by the *śabda* "cow"; and (3) there is a predicate relation in which *śabda* and *artha* are dominated and appropriated by the *jñāna* "cow."

Vyāsa finds that the psychological cause of this mixed-up perception of the true meaning is twofold. On the one hand, there is the distortion caused by the *saṁskāras* of *saṅketa* (conventional word use in previous lives), discussed above, and resulting in the universally experienced error of type (2) *vikalpa*. On the other hand, there are the cognitive inferences (*anumānas*) based upon the *artha*, made by one's own imaginative thinking or heard from the traditional schools of thought (*darśanas*). Such *anumāna*-dominated hearing would seem to be an error of type (3) with the erroneous element being the "slanting" or "coloring" given the *sphoṭa* by the doctrinal presuppositions of the particular *darśana* heard. Although not elucidated by either Vyāsa or Vācaspati, the type (1) situation, in which the *artha* predominates, would seem to be closest to true perception yet still erroneous due to its predicate relations with the other two types. Such predicate relations would be experienced because of the finite structural individuations of consciousness through which the speech is necessarily heard (i.e., the organ of hearing, *manas*, *prāṇa*, *śabda-tanmātra*, etc.) in ordinary states of consciousness. These types of *vikalpa* are therefore shown to be the psychological processes producing the high error perception that characterizes the verbal, or *vaikharī*, level of hearing. To such high-error-level perception Yoga applies the technical term *savitarkā*, which means indistinct concentration (*samādhi*) of the consciousness.

As the concentrated perception of the word is gradually purified or freed from memory (*saṅketa*) and the predicate relations of inference (*anumāna*), the consciousness state approaches what Bharthari calls *madhyamā vāk*. This is the inner hearing aspect of the complete communication circle the *sphoṭa* forms in its "vibratory movement" from the *buddhi* of the speaker to the *buddhi* of the hearer. In the *Vākyapadīya* commentaries, it is described as having the *ahaṁkāra*, or ego, as its only substratum and having sequence present but only in a very subtle fashion. *Dhvani* and *artha* are still distinct and the order of words is present. Although sequence or predicate relations are suppressed, they are said to be accompanied by a distinct functioning of *prāṇa*.[41] Whereas in the speaking act the psychomotor *prāṇa*, or breath, functions served to individuate the *sphoṭa* pattern through the coordination of the *śabda-tanmātra* and vocal organ, the process is reversed in hearing with *prāṇa* and *manas* working to reintegrate the gross differentiations of the *sphoṭa* pattern at the ear level into the less differentiated vibration patterns of the *śabda tanmātra*, *manas*, and *ahaṁkāra*. As the more integrated heights of *madhyamā vāk* are realized, the overall preponderance of *sattva* in the *sphoṭa* vibration pattern correspondingly increases until a clearer perception of the unified *sphoṭa* occurs.

A kind of idealized or criterion description of *madhyamā* in its purest form is offered by the Yoga analysis of *savicāra*, or meditative, *samādhi*.[42] In *savicāra* the intensity of concentration is such that the *sattva* is so transparent that the *artha*, or true meaning, of the given *sphoṭa* stands revealed in the mind (*antaḥkāraṇa*) with little distortion or obscuration. On the subjective (*sattva*) side, the distortion decreases as the integration of the heard *sphoṭa* moves from the high *rajas*-low *sattva* ratio of the *manas* and senses to the low *rajas*-high *sattva* ratio of the *ahaṁkāra*. On the objective (*tamas*) side, the overall obscuration of the *sphoṭa*-patterned consciousness state decreases as the *rajas* activation of the *śabda tanmātra* becomes less and less until the state of pure potential is approached. Vyāsa describes the *savicāra* state as being composed of the essences of all the gross particularizations of the *sphoṭa* pattern. Vācaspati notes that just as the gross atoms (at the *vaikharī* level) are patterned by the *manas* and *prāṇa* into a whole by a single effort of consciousness, so also in the *savicāra* state the subtle electron-like *tanmātras* are patterned by the *prāṇa*—although less *prāṇa* than at the *vaikharī* level—and the *antaḥkaraṇa* into the same whole by a single effort of consciousness.

The distortions still found at the *savicāra* level of inner hearing include notions of time, place, and causation. But characteristics associated with the hearing of the gross sound (dialect, speed of speaking, emotional colorations by voice, timbre, etc.) will have virtually all dropped away in the *savicāra citta*. The influence of *saṅketa saṁskāras* (memory traces of conventional word usage), while not entirely absent, will be greatly reduced. Far more powerful will be the intensifying of the *artha* aspect of the *sattva citta* due to magnet-like attraction exerted by the pure *saṁskāra* series of the *buddhitattva sphoṭa* upon the "approaching" and integrating manifestation of the *sphoṭa* pattern within the listener's consciousness.

Although the above Yoga analysis provides a psychological description of the meditative, or *madhyamā*, *vāk* and satisfies the primary task of the psychological interpretation, the secondary question of how one's ordinary *vaikharī* perception of *vāk*, which is in the confused *savitarkā* state of consciousness, can be raised to a higher level, has yet to be answered. This second answer is especially important if Bhartṛhari is correct in his observation that in many people, owing to poor word usage in their previous lives, the divine *vāk* (in its pristine state as the pure *saṁskāra* series of Īśvara's *sattva*) has become badly mixed up with corrupt word forms. And since both the divine and the corrupt forms are being handed down to us in our inherent *vāsanās*, some means of purifying one's *vāk* is required in order to avoid being trapped forever at the *vaikharī* level.[43] Should this happen, not only would we be prevented from the earthly happiness and merit that result from the correct use of words, but we would also suffer the endless pain engendered by never being able to achieve the ultimate bliss of *mokṣa*, which comes from the realization of oneness with *Śabdabrahman*. Bhartṛhari clearly assumes the practical possibility of such a purification of one's *vāk*. Although he does not describe the process required, he technically designates it as *śabdapūrvayoga*.

ŚABDAPŪRVAYOGA AS INTERPRETED BY THE *YOGA SŪTRAS*

If one is fortunate enough to be born as a sage, as a result of the cumulative effect of good word use in previous lives, little more than continued practice of *vairāgya*—the turning away of the mind from all forms of worldly attachment—and *abhysa*—the habitual steadying of the mind in concentration upon the Vedic *sphoṭa*—is required to ensure ascent to Śabdabrahman.[44] But before the ordinary person can attempt such advanced *vairāgya* and *abhyāsa*, his habitually distracted state of mind, owing to lack of concentration and the obscuring habit patterns of bad word usage (*vāsanās*), must be overcome. To this end the *Yoga Sūtras* offer some specific techniques that may well have been what Bhartṛhari had in mind as *śabdapūrvayoga*. According to Vyāsa, these Yoga techniques function simply by removing the obstacles (i.e., the *vāsanās*, or habit patterns, of bad word usage) that are preventing consciousness from flowing toward *mokṣa* under the motive force of its own inherent teleology. Yoga psychology maintains that in itself consciousness (*citta*) is always attempting to move toward *mokṣa*. Therefore, all that the specific Yoga techniques do is to remove the obstructions within the mind, and consciousness then passes naturally into the state of *mokṣa*.[45]

In *Yoga Sūtra* 11: 29, Patañjali lists eight Yoga techniques or practices (*yogāṅga*). They are *yama*, or restraints; *niyama*, or disciplines; *āsanas*, or body postures; *prāṇāyāma*, or regulation of breath; *pratyāhāra*, or freedom of the mind from sensory domination by external objects; *dhāraṇā*, or concentration; *dhyāna*, or Yogic meditation; and *samādhi*, or trance. These classic Yoga disciplines will be examined in relation to Bhartṛhari's concept of *śabdapūrvayoga*.

Although Patañjali lists five *yamas*, or self-restraints, which when practiced will remove the gross impurities obstructing the perception of *sphoṭa* in ordinary minds, from the point of view of *śabdapūrvayoga* it is the discipline of *satya*, or truthfulness, that commands special attention. *Satya* is the conformity of one's speech and mind (*citta vṛtti*) with the thing itself. Word and thought must conform with the facts that have been seen, heard, and inferred. Vyāsa points out that since the function of speech is to communicate one's understanding to others, therefore it must contain no illusion, nor should it create illusion in others if it is true speech (*vāk*). This *vāk* is for the benefit of all beings, not for their injury. In this regard, Manu is quoted: "Utter what is beneficial to others; do not utter what is true but injurous to others . . . therefore, after careful enquiry one should speak the truth which will be beneficial to all beings."[46]

In addition to speaking the truth, there are the powerful cleansing and mind-controlling practices of *svādhyāya*. *Svādhyāya*, or concentrated study (*Yoga Sūtra* II: 32), includes both the recital of passages of scripture, and the repetition of *mantras* such as *AUM*. *Study* here implies not only reading the scripture for its rational content but also saying it meditatively. Without any attempt at rational analysis, one simply repeats the verse over and over so as to let the revelatory power inherent within it work upon one's consciousness. In addition to repeating scriptural verses in this fashion, one should also chant the sacred syllable *AUM*. The more one repeats such verbalizations of the *ṛṣis*, the more power they have to break through the veiling ignorance of one's mind so as to evoke or reveal the Divine Word that is within. In terms of the "energy vibration" analogy used previously to describe the hearing of the spoken word, the process would be as follows. Concentrated repetitions reinforce the "*sattvic* vibrations" which the spoken Vedic words induce within the mental organ (*antaḥkararṇa*), resulting in a powerful sympathetic "vibration" deep within the *paśyantī*, or highest level of consciousness, until the pure *sphoṭa* is revealed in a flash of insight.

This conception of study aims at freeing one's mind of obstructions and distractions and simply allowing the power of the Divine Word to work within one's consciousness. Rather than doing the thinking and revealing the truth by one's own effort, as is the case in rational analysis, here one is quieting one's own thinking and allowing the Divine Word, which is both immanent within consciousness and externally presented as the authoritative scriptural revelation, itself to speak. While this kind of "study" until recently was virtually unknown in modern Western life, it was present in the medieval West and is currently being rediscovered in contemporary movements such as Transcendental Meditation and the new interest in Christian Monastic Contemplation.[47]

As *vāk*, including both external speaking and internal thinking, becomes more meditative, there is a reduction in all gross psychomotor activity.[48] In Yoga this internalization of concentration is fostered by the three aids of body postures (*āsanas*), breath control (*prāṇāyāma*), and withdrawal of senses (*pratyahāra*). The taking up of a stable posture, or *āsana*, is not complete until it can be maintained without any mental effort so that all possible movements of the body are restrained, thus freeing consciousness from gross *prāṇa* activity and assisting in stabilizing the subtle *prāṇa* required for *madhyamā vāk*.[49] A practical criterion is given whereby the Yogin can test himself. Mastery of *āsanas* is indicated when the Yogin can remain unaffected by the pairs of opposites, such as heat and cold, while meditating upon his verse, or *mantra*.[50]

As another aid to *śabdapūrvayoga*, the devotee must further control the *vaikharī*, or ordinary expression of speech and thought, by the practice of *prāṇāyāma* (controlled respiration). In Yoga Sutra II: 49 and 50, *Prāṇāyāma* is defined as the practice of pausing after each deep inhalation and each deep exhalation. When practiced in conjunction with *āsana*, a high degree of external stability and control is achieved over involvements of consciousness in the gross sequences that characterize the manifestation of *vakharī vāk*. As Bhartṛhari observes, at the *madhyamā* level the cognition of *vāk* is chiefly associated with the internal mental organ (*antaḥkaraṇa*) and not with the organs of gross articulation or hearing, and therefore the kind of *prāṇa* required is very subtle. By using various specified methods of measurement, the Yogin can determine the length of pauses he is achieving and compare them against the established standards: *mātrā*, or instant (the time taken to snap the fingers after turning the hand over the knee three times), first or mild *udghāta* (thirty-six such *mātrās*), second or moderate *udghāta* (first *udghāta* doubled), and third or intense *udghāta* (first *udghāta* tripled). A special fourth kind of *prāṇāyāma* is achieved by applying the Yogic psychological principle of counteracting unwanted tendencies by the forceful practice of their opposites. In this case, the breath is drawn in forcibly when it has a tendency to go out, and thrown out forcibly when it has a tendency to go in. By such negative practice plus the three easier kinds of restraint, breathing becomes so inhibited that it may virtually cease for long periods. The purpose of this practice is said to be the destruction of the impurities, such as delusions caused by traces of corrupt word usage, from consciousness until it becomes so luminous, or sattvic, that clear perception of the *sphoṭa* becomes possible.[51] Only then is the mind judged to be truly fit for *dhyāna*, or "fixed concentration." As Eliade observes, a remark of Bhoja states clearly the underlying principle: "All the functions of the organs being preceded by that of respiration—there being always a connection between respiration and consciousness in their respective functions—respiration, when all the functions of the organs are suspended, realizes concentration of consciousness on a single object."[52] This principle, that there is a direct connection between respiration and mental states, is fundamental for Yoga.

A further aid to turning the flow of consciousness away from the gross manifestations of uttered speech and toward the *sphoṭa's* internal *artha* (meaning) aspect is the Yoga practice of *pratyāhāra*. *Pratyāhāra* is defined as the disciplined withdrawal of the senses from their preoccupation with external manifestations so as to become focused with all of consciousness in single-pointed contemplation of the internal *artha*. Vyāsa offers the analogy that, just as when the king bee (queen bee in the West) settles down, all the other bees follow, so, when consciousness is restricted and concentrated, the sense organs are also withdrawn and concentrated. This is *pratyāhāra*, which, along with the practice of *āsanas* and *prāṇāyāma*, results in control over the *vaikharī*, or external expression of *vāk*.

In the above discussion it has been shown how the practices detailed by the *Yoga Sūtras* purify consciousness to the level of single-pointedness (*ekāgratā*). This Yoga analysis would seem to correspond with Bhartṛhari's basic requirements for *śabdapūrvayoga*—the rising above the gross expression of *prāṇa* and the cutting of the knots that bring about the differentiation of *vāk*.[53]

The last three practices, described as the direct aids to Yoga, are: *dhāraṇā*, or fixed concentration; *dhyāna*, or yogic meditation; and *samādhi*, or trance contemplation. They represent three stages of the same process, which is given the technical name *saṁyama* (perfected contemplation).[54] For the practice of *śabdapūrvayoga*, *dhāraṇā* would be the fixed concentration of consciousness upon the *artha*, or meaning, of the *sphoṭa*. Dasgupta helpfully clarifies the necessary relationship between *dhāraṇā* and *pratyāhāra* (withdrawal of senses). *Dhāraṇā* and *pratyāhāra* must be practiced together as conjoint means for achieving the same end. *Dhāraṇā* without *pratyāhāra* or *pratyāhāra* without *dhāraṇā* would both be a fruitless endeavor.[55] Vijñāna Bhikṣu suggests that in terms of elapsed time, *dhāraṇā* must last as long as twelve *prāṇāyāmas*.[56]

Dhyāna is the continuance or uninterrupted flow of fixed concentration upon *artha* in the stream of consciousness.[57] It is the continuation of the mental effort to clearly perceive the *sphoṭa*. Vijñāna Bhikṣu indicates that in terms of elapsed time, *dhyāna* may be thought of as lasting as long as twelve *dharaṇās*, which would equal one hundred forty-four *prāṇāyāmas*. Mastery at this *madhyamā* level of *vāk* is indicated by the lack of intrusion of any other mental state (*citta-vṛtti*) during this period of meditation.

Samādhi, or trance contemplation, occurs when the *dhyāna* loses its subject-object distinction. As Vyāsa puts it, when fixed concentration shines forth only in the form of the object being contemplated and empty of all duality, that is *samādhi*.[58] Vācaspati further clarifies the point as follows. A *kalpanā* or two-termed relation is a distinction between the concentration and the object upon which it is fixed. *Dhāraṇā* and *dhyāna* exhibit such subject-object distinction. However, all duality is absent in *samādhi*, where the mind has fused itself with or become one with the object. In this state there is no self-awareness but only a direct intuition—knowing by becoming one with the object. For *śabdapūrvayoga* this would mark the transition from the dualistic experience of *sphoṭa* as *dhvani* and *artha*, grossly manifested at the *vaikharī* level and subtly manifested at the *madhyamā* level, to the unitary perception of the *sphoṭa*, which characterizes the *pratibhā* of the *paśyantī* level of *vāk*. It is this *paśyantī* state of *sphoṭa samādhi* that provides the psychological process by which the *śabda* devotee may make his ascent toward *mokṣa*—union with *Śabdabrahman*. At the lower levels of *vaikharī* and *madhyamā*, however, the correct use of words through practices such as *satya* helps to produce spiritual merit (*dharma*), which makes certain the attainment of happiness here and beyond. But for the ultimate end, correct usage alone is not enough. When the lower practices (*yogāṅgas*) are combined with the higher *samādhi* forms, *śabdapūrvayoga* then opens the way to the ultimate end and the realization of *mokṣa*.

Samādhi is the goal of the *śabdapūrvayoga*, and all the Yoga practices must work together for its achievement. It cannot be achieved unless, as the Yogin tries to withdraw his or her senses and focus the mind, potential obstructions arising from the unsteadiness of the body and the mind are controlled by *āsana* and *prāṇāyāma*. And then only gradually, through the steadying of the mind on one *sphoṭa*, does consciousness (*citta*) begin to flow evenly without any disruption. Finally, the mind even ceases to think that it is thinking the *sphoṭa* itself. Although, theoretically, the last three stages are separated, Patañjali makes clear that in practice *dhāraṇā*, *dhyāna*, and *samādhi* are all part of the same process of which the last one is perfection. Success is indicated by the shining forth of *prajñā* (insight or direct perception of the *sphoṭa*), and is the *paśyantī* level of *vāk*.[59]

Throughout the *Vākyapadīya* analysis of the levels of *vāk*, it seems clear that Bhartṛhari's concept is that these levels are heuristic levels on a continuum rather than discrete hierarchial stages. The same sort of heuristic continuum is also envisaged in the Yoga analysis of the various levels of *samādhi*.[60] This means that within the *paśyantī pratibhā* there will be degrees of clearness in the unitary perception of *sphoṭa*. It is fitting, therefore, that in the *Yoga Sūtras*, when *samādhi* is being analyzed in its nondualistic or *pratibhā* state, two qualities of *prajñā* are described: *nirvitarka*, or gross *pratibhā* of the *sphoṭa*, and *nirvicāra*, or subtle *pratibhā* of the *sphoṭa*.

Nirvitarka, or gross perception of the *sphoṭa*, occurs when the *samādhi* is freed from memory, the conventional usage of *śabda*, and the predicate relations of *jñāna* by inference or association, allowing the thing-itself (*svarūpa*) to shine forth in itself alone. In this stage the *svarūpa* (*sphoṭa*) is directly intuited as having just that form which it has in itself and nothing more. *Citta* has become one with the object so that the object no longer appears as an object of consciousness.[61] The duality of subject and object is overcome, leaving only the steady transformation of *citta* in the form of the object of its contemplation. Here the *samādhi* knowledge, or *prajñā*, is an outgrowth from the *savitarka samādhi*. It is of the grosser *vaikharī* manifestation of the *sphoṭa* as perceived in its formal pattern or unity through the senses.

Nirvicāra samādhi develops naturally from the meditative concentration (*savicāra*) that was previously found to characterize *madhyamā vāk*. When, by constant *śabdapūrvayoga*, the mind becomes so much identified with the subtle aspects of the *savicāra samādhi* that notions of time, place, and causality disappear, and the *antaḥkaraṇa* becomes one with the *sattvic sphoṭa*, that is, *nirvicāra*.[62] In this *samādhi* state, the *śabda* Yogin's *citta* becomes so purified that the *prajñā* obtained is perfectly pure and considered to be absolute knowledge of the *sphoṭa*. It is the final, clear, no-error perception of the *sphoṭa* at the opposite end of the hearer's continuum from the high-error initial experiences of the phonemes at the *vaikharī* level. This *nirvicāra samādhi*, which is Patañjali's highest *samprajñāta* or "seeded" stage, seems equivalent to Bhartṛhari's *viśiṣṭopahita*, or highest *pratibhā*.[63] It is the same process by which the *ṛṣis* cognize the Vedas, but unlike the more ordinary *śabda* Yogin, the great sages are said to have been able to directly perceive the noumenal *sphoṭa* without having to go through the process of errors. The *prajñā*, or knowledge revealed by the direct perception of the *sphoṭa*, is described as having a twofold character: it gives the special or true knowledge of the word, and it gives the power to act in accordance with that knowledge.[64] It is through both of these capacities that the *pratibhā* perception of *sphoṭa* provides the means for *mokṣa* realization. From the Yoga viewpoint, this situation is described in a more technical psychological fashion, as follows. When the *śabda* Yogin remains in the concentrated insight of the *nirvicāra* state, the ongoing impact of this insight (*prajñā*) upon consciousness effectively restricts the emergence of any remaining negative *saṁskāras*. By such *śabdapūrvayoga*, any remaining obstacles are removed, and the inherent telos within consciousness itself finds *mokṣa*, or oneness with *Śabdabrahman*.

4

Yoga in the *Vairāgya-Śataka* of Bhartṛhari

In addition to establishing himself in the classical Indian tradition as a grammarian and a metaphysician, and having established a basis for literary criticism, Bhartṛhari is also well known for his Sanskrit poetry. In popular Indian thought, Bhartṛhari is identified as a king who was discouraged by the inconstancy of women and was thus led to renounce the world of sensuous experience. One of his verses recounts the experience with the depth and compactness that characterizes his poetry.

> She who is the constant object of my thought
> Is indifferent to me,
> Is desirous of another man,
> Who in his turn adores some other woman,
> But this woman takes delight in me . . .
> Damn her! Damn him! The God of love!
> The other woman! And Myself![1]

Tradition seems to have consistently maintained that Bhartṛhari, the poet, was the same Bhartṛhari who composed the *Vākyapadīya* and a commentary on the Mahābhāṣya of Patañjali. This ancient tradition identifying Bhartṛhari the poet with Bhartṛhari the grammarian was called into question by scholars writing around 1900 (e.g., M. R. Kale[2]) and more recently by D. D. Kosambi.[3] Kosambi's argument, however, although meticulously researched, depends for its strength on the Chinese pilgrim I-tsing's suggestion that the Bhartṛhari of the *Vākyapadīya* was a Buddhist. Since Bhartṛhari the poet shows no trace of Buddhism, Kosambi felt that there must be two different Bhartṛharis. However, the contents of that work are thoroughly Brāhmanical in nature. This, plus the dating of Bhartṛhari as prior to the fifth century CE (on the basis of Bhartṛhari quotations in the works of Diṅnāga), has led recent scholarship to re-examine the identity thesis of the classical tradition.[4] Not only does the author of this book adopt the traditional viewpoint on this question, but it is suggested that Bhartṛhari's assumption of Patañjali's classical Yoga in the *Vākyapadīya* (see chapter 2) also occurs in his poetry and is further evidence for the identity thesis. Thus, in addition to introducing the reader to Bhartṛhari's poetry, this chapter takes as its point of focus the Yoga psychology assumed in the verses of the *Vairāgya-Śataka*.

BHARTṚHARI THE POET

Bhartṛhari's *Vairāgya-Śataka*, or "Hundred Verses on Renunciation," is a poem of ancient India that may still be found upon the lips of Indians today. The *Vairāgya* is the third in a trilogy of poems by Bhartṛhari, each one hundred verses in length. The other two poems are entitled the *Nīti-Śataka* (on politics and ethics), and the *Śṛṅgāra-Śataka* (on passionate love). The fact that these very old poems are still a part of the consciousness of contemporary India is one important reason for their study. Perhaps even more important, however, is the way in which both the world-transcending ideals of Indian religion and the Indian experience of sensual love are held in tension within the poems. While the West has identified both full enjoyment of the senses and the rigorous renunciation of the senses with India, most often these two aspects have remained quite disconnected. Bhartṛhari's poetry, especially the *Vairāgya*, includes both the sensuous and the sense-renouncing aspects of the Indian consciousness in a way that presents a rounded exposure of India to the modern reader. In the *Vairāgya*, Bhartṛhari presents us with the creative tension between a profound attraction to sensual beauty and the yearning for liberation from it. From this study valuable insight may be gained as to how Indian religion, art, and culture can be at once so sensuous and so spiritual.[5]

A *śataka*, in Sanskrit poetry, is a hundred detached verses having a common theme such as *vairāgya*, or renunciation. Each four-line verse is intended to convey a complete mood, or *rasa*, and to stand on its own as an aesthetic entity. Bhartṛhari's verses are characterized by the amount of complex thought and detail that he compresses into a simple metrical pattern. Barbara Miller, who has successfully translated his verses into English, suggests that "the stanzas may be compared to the miniature paintings which illustrate the manuscripts of medieval India. Profusion is forced into a miniature mould; the mould is then expanded by exploiting the suggestive overtones (*dhvani*) of words and images."[6]

In India the life of an individual was ideally divided into four different stages: the student stage, the householder stage, the withdrawal from worldly life into the forest, and finally the stage of the wandering hermit or holy man. Bhartṛhari's poems reflect one's spiritual development through these stages. The *Nīti-Śataka* comments on the life of worldly possessions and political power. The *Śṛṅgāra-Śataka* sensitively evokes the erotic mood of love, which, along with the pursuit of worldly possessions and power, characterizes the householder stage of life. But even within this stage there are seeds of discontent that motivate the sensitive soul toward the withdrawal and spiritual discipline of the final two stages. Bhartṛhari's poetry captures this discontent in its revulsion against the sordidness of worldly life and in its awareness that the delights of passionate love are at once beautiful and enslaving.

> A man may tread the righteous path,
> Be master of his senses,
> Retire in timidity
> Or cling to modest ways—only until
> The seductive arrow-glances of amorous women
> Fall on his heart,
> Glances drawn to her ear,
> Shot from the bow of her brow,
> And winged by long black lashes.
> The path which leads beyond
> Your bounds, Saṁsāra,
> Would be less treacherous
> Were it not for intoxicating glances
> Waylaying us at every turn. (*Śṛṅgāra-Śataka, slokas* 35 and 43)

In the end it is through the renunciation described in the *Vairāgya-Śataka* that release from such worldly desires may be achieved. The *Vairāgya* presents a poetic picture of the renunciation of the last two stages of life. Here the ascetic finds the dispassionate tranquillity of the forest as he passes his days in meditation on the bank of a mountain river. Release from the worldly life of sense enslavement is accomplished through the discipline of Yoga, and this therefore is the dominant theme throughout the *Vairāgya-Śataka.*

In chapter 3 of this book it was suggested that the Yoga psychology assumed by Bhartṛhari in his *Vākyapadīya* is the Yoga of Patañjali. Bhartṛhari's *Vairāgya* is also firmly based on that same Yoga, which begins with a diagnosis of the states of consciousness making up ordinary human experience (*kleśas*) and then details the eight steps to release (*yogāṇgas*).

DIAGNOSIS OF THE HUMAN CONDITION

In his analysis of the states of consciousness (*citta vṛtti*) Patañjali finds that all ordinary experience may be divided into five types: ignorance (*avidyā*), egoism (*asmitā*), passion (*rāga*), disgust (*dveṣa*) and clinging to life (*abhiniveśa*).[7] On close examination, each of these is found to end in suffering; therefore they are classed as *kleśas*, or constantly changing painful states of consciousness. Patañjali's analysis brings out philosophical and psychological dimensions that parallel descriptions found in Bhartṛhari's poetry. The poetic parallels may well convey a more comprehensive understanding of the Yogic experience than the *sūtras* and commentaries alone can provide. It has long been the contention of Indian literary critics that the aesthetic consciousness (*rasa-dhvani*) evoked by poetry transcends the dry and partial descriptions of the scholars.

Avidyā is the beginningless ignorance that obscures the inherent omniscience of consciousness from view. Patañjali describes *avidyā* as the root *kleśa* of *citta.*[8] *Avidyā* is defined philosophically as the taking of the noneternal (*anitya*), the impure (*asuchi*), the painful (*duḥkha*), and the not-self (*anātman*) to be the eternal, the pure, the pleasurable, and the self.[9] Through the Yogic analysis, every kind of worldly experience, with its sensual attachment to objects, is in the end seen to give only temporary pleasure. Due to the insatiability of desire, sensual indulgence only results in a constant craving for more. Thus, for the Yogin, every pleasure is seen as a pain in the making.

In the poetic vision of the *Vairāgya*, *avidyā* also appears as the root of suffering. In *sloka* 18, *avidyā* is depicted as an insect that stupidly jumps into the fire or a fish that through ignorance takes the baited hook.[10] The human being, however, with the power of intelligent discrimination should avoid the hook, but the power of ignorant passion is so deluding that he or she greedily eats the bait. Even the ravages of time cannot remove us from the grip of *avidyā*.

My face is graven with wrinkles
My head is marked with grey,
My limbs are withered and feeble—
My craving alone keeps its youth. (*sloka* 8)

Asmitā, or egoism, results from the taking of one's body and thoughts to be one's true self (*ātman*).[11] In *sloka* 70, Bhartṛhari captures the meaning intended by Patañjali.

You descend to nether worlds,
You traverse the sky,
You roam the horizon
With restless mobility my mind!
Why do you never, even in error,
Stumble on what is pure
And the true part of yourself,
That Brahman, through which
You would reach your final bliss?

It is from such deluded egoism that *rāga* springs forth. *Rāga*, says Patañjali, is a thirst for pleasure by one who has previously experienced pleasures (in this or previous lives) and remembers them.[12] The poet brings out the full fury of *rāga* by comparing the condition of an ignorant man with that of the enlightened Lord Śiva. "Ordinary persons when they give themselves up to enjoyment, lose all control and become slaves to them; so even when satiety comes they cannot detach themselves. But Śiva, who has [purged the ignorance from his mind], is unaffected by them."[13]

Dveṣa, or aversion, is the opposite of *rāga*. It also springs from the ego-sense, which having experienced and remembered pain feels anxiety for its removal.[14] For the sensitive poetic mind, such remembrance is indeed painful and urges one toward the Yogic path of release.

Abandon the depths of sensuous chaos,
That prison of torment!
The course reaching beyond toward bliss

Can instantly allay all pain.
Initiate then a peaceful mood!
Renounce your gamboling unsteady ways!
Forsake the ephemeral mundane passions!
Rest placid now, my thoughts! (*sloka* 63)

But such anxiety and aversion are often countered by the strong impulsion within ignorant egoism for its own survival. *Abhiniveśa*, shrinking from death and clinging to life, is found by Patañjali to be rooted in *avidyā* and to spring from egoism. It is an endless craving for one's self. In an image remarkably similar to Yeats's "An aged man is but a paltry thing, a tattered coat upon a stick,"[15] Bhartṛhari describes the body that "can raise itself but slowly on the staff" yet "still startles at the thought of dissolution by death."[16] Patañjali remarks that this fear of death is found in both the stupid and the wise and gives evidence that the round of birth and rebirth (*saṁsāra*) must have been experienced by all.[17]

Within the constant circle of *saṁsāra*, both Patañjali and Bhartṛhari describe consciousness by analogy to the flow of a river. In the *Yoga Sūtras*, the changing movement of mental states (*citta-vṛttis*) is said to be like a river whose flow is in two directions: toward good and toward evil.[18] Within itself, pure *citta* has an inherent tendency to flow in the direction of good, and this can never be totally lost. But *citta* is polluted by the *karmic* seeds of past thoughts and actions, and these make consciousness flow in the opposite direction, creating the whirlpool of existence called *saṁsāra*. When one has dammed up the flow of *citta* toward objects seen (women, food, drink, power, etc.) by *vairāgya*, and opened the flood gates toward *mokṣa*, or release from *saṁsāra* by practice in discriminative knowledge, then *citta* will flow toward good.[19] In poetic terms the same complex situation is described by Bhartṛhari:

Hope is a river
Whose water is desire,
Whose waves are craving.
Passions are crocodiles,
Conjectures are birds
Destroying the tree of resolve.
Anxiety carves a deep ravine
And makes the whirlpool of delusion
Makes it difficult to ford.
Let ascetics who cross
To the opposite shore
Exult in their purified minds, (*sloka* 10)

Such is the diagnosis of our ordinary mental state with its polluting *kleśas*. Now the question arises as to what treatment can be taken so that the pollution may be purged, the whirlpool stilled, and the peaceful purity of mind realized. The treatment offered by both Bhartṛhari and Patañjali is the renunciation of worldly desires by the concentration of *citta* through Yoga.

TREATMENT OF THE HUMAN CONDITION

Patañjali states that the practice of the *yogāṇgas*, or steps to Yoga, results in the purging of *karmic* impurities from the stream of consciousness so that its inherent omniscience may shine forth. The purifying action of the *yogāṇgas* is likened to an ax splitting off the offending *kleśas* from *citta*.[20] The eight steps in the practice of yoga listed by Patañjali[21] have been introduced in earlier chapters.

The first step on the path of Yogic treatment is *yama*. Patañjali lists five *yamas*, or self-disciplines, which when practiced will remove the gross *karmic* impurities from our ordinary mental state. *Ahiṁsā*, or noninjury, is the root *yama* and requires nonviolence in thought as well as action.[22] The test for having mastered *ahimṣā* is that the peacefulness of one's *citta* will affect all other persons and animals within one's presence so that they give up their natural hostility to one another. The cobra and mongoose will lie down together beside the Yogin.[23] Or as Bhartṛhari puts it, "Blessed are those who live in mountain caves, meditating on Brahman, the Supreme Light, while birds devoid of fear perch on their laps and drink the tear drops of bliss that they shed in meditation."[24] Other than *ahimṣā*, the *yamas* include the practices of *satya*, or truthfulness; *asteya*, or nonstealing; *brahmacarya*, or control of sexual desire; and *aparigraha*, or the absence of avarice. These are effectively captured in a verse from the *Nīti-Śataka, sloka* 3:

> Refrain from taking life,
> Never envy other men's wealth,
> Speak words of truth,
> Give timely alms within your means . . .
> Dam the torrent of your craving,
> Do reverence before the venerable,
> And bear compassion for all creatures . . .

Together with the above restraints, the Yogin must observe a series of *niyamas*, or positive practices of body and mind. *Samtoṣa* is described by Patañjali as the absence of desire for more than the necessities of life.[25] It is sensitively captured in Bhartṛhari's poetry.

> I dwell content in the hermit's dress of bark,
> While you luxuriate in silken splendor.
> Still, my contentment is equal to yours;
> Disparity's guise is deceiving.
> Now let him be called a pauper
> Who bears insatiable greed;
> But when a mind rests content,
> What can it mean to be "wealthy" or "poor"? (*sloka* 53)

Tapas, or the practice of austerities, consists in bearing with equanimity the pairs of opposites such as heat and cold, hunger and thirst.[26] The poet concurs: "Nothing is good for the wise in this world excepting the practice of austerities!"[27] For Patañjali,

Īśvarapranidhana is the offering up of all actions to the Lord, so that all work is done not for one's own self but for God.[28] For Bhartṛhari, the vision of the unrelenting approach of death leads him to take refuge in the Lord alone.[29] *Svādhyāya*, or the study of Vedic texts and the repetition of syllables (e.g., AUM) that lead to release, is revered by Patañjali[30] and Bhartṛhari. The poet maintains that while other vows may lead to worldly prosperity, the repetition of Vedic vows results in spiritual peace.[31]

In *sūtras* II: 33 and 34, Patañjali states a most important psychological insight (today called "behavior therapy") which seems to be a basic assumption for the practice of Yoga in all Indian systems. When a yogin while performing his *yogāṅgas* finds himself beset by doubts or desires, he should counteract such perverse thoughts (*vitarkas*) by the cultivation of their opposites (*pratipaksa bhāvanā*). Bhartṛhari not only captures this insight but at the same time seems to identify this difficulty as being a particular weakness of the poet.

> Her breasts, those fleshy protuberances,
> Are compared to golden bowls;
> Her face, a vile receptacle of phlegm,
> Is likened to the moon;
> Her thighs, dank with urine, are said
> To rival the elephant's trunk.
> Mark how this despicable form
> Is flourished by the poets, (*sloka* 16)

Of course this kind of "cultivating of opposites" can be practiced on the male body with equal success if the Yogin happens to be a woman. Underlying this practical psychology is the theoretical analysis of how actualized *karmas* create a potency, or *saṁskāra*, for the repetition of the same act or thought to be laid down in the subconscious *citta* where the appropriate moment for a new actualization of the *karma* is awaited. Such habitual behavior or thought patterns are self-reinforcing in nature and can be broken only by the self-conscious act of creating sufficient opposing *karmas* so that even the unactualized *saṁskāras* will be rendered impotent.[32]

Āsanas, or body postures, are prescribed by Patañjali to control the restless activity of one's body—a necessary prerequisite to the controlling of one's mind. The *sūtra* describes the kind of posture required as being stable, motionless, and easy to maintain.[33] With all possible body movements restrained, the *citta* is left free for its efforts toward concentration. Toward the end of the *Vairāgya-Śataka* we find the poet adopting an *āsana*: "Sitting in peaceful posture, during the nights when all sounds are stilled into silence . . . fearful of the miseries of birth and death, crying aloud 'Śiva, Śiva, Śiva. . . .'"[34] Along with the practice of stable sitting, the Yogin has to master controlled breathing, or *prāṇāyāma*. Although this practice is not specifically mentioned in the poem, it is clearly assumed in the repeated urgings toward a quiet and calm mind.[35] Regulation of breathing is based on the principle that there is a direct connection between the rate of respiration and mental states. This is known to the modern neurophysiologist and is easily observable by any layperson. In states of emotional arousal (especially of the passionate variety so clearly examined in Bhartṛhari's *Śṛṅgāra-Śataka*) respiration is uneven and fast, while in one who is concentrating it becomes rhythmical and slow. In such concentration there is also *pratyāhāra*, or withdrawal of the senses from attachment to external objects, and instead the inward focusing of the sense organs and all of *citta* on the *ātman*, or true self. As Bhartṛhari puts it, "Desist, O heart, from the troublous labyrinth of sense-objects; take that path of (highest) good which is capable of bringing about in a moment the destruction of endless troubles; get thee to the state of thy *Ātman*."[36]

The last three *yogāṅgas* (*dhāraṇā*, or fixed concentration; *dhyāna*, or Yogic meditation; and *samādhi*, or trance concentration) are not easily separated. Patañjali says that they represent three stages of the same process in which the subject-object duality of ordinary cognition is gradually purified until "oneness with the object" (knowing by becoming one with) is achieved.[37] As Vyāsa puts it, when fixed concentration shines forth only in the form of the object being contemplated and empty of all duality, that is *samādhi*.[38] In this state there is no self-awareness but only direct intuition; *citta*, or consciousness, knows by fusing itself with the object. And for both the *Yoga Sūtras* and the *Vairāgya-Śataka*, the intended object is the Lord (Īśvara for Patañjali; Śiva for Bhartṛhari).

> Purge your delusion
> Find joy in moon-crested Śiva,
> Dwell in devotion, my thoughts,
> On the banks of the heavenly river! . . . (*sloka* 64)

For Bhartṛhari, through intense devotional concentration on Brahman as the Lord, a final stage of transcendent consciousness is reached. At this rarefied height, words are quite inadequate. While useful in raising us to this height (see chapter 2), individual words must ultimately be transcended. Patañjali technically terms the experience *nirvicāra samādhi*. It is the state achieved when by constant practice the mind loses the notions of time, place, and causality and becomes one with the essence of its object of concentration.[39] Bhartṛhari, through the poetic form, perhaps comes close to expressing this experience:

> O Earth, my mother! O Wind, my father! O Fire, my friend! O Water, my good relative! O Sky, my brother! here is my last salutation to you with clasped hands! Having cast away Infatuation with its wonderful power, by means of an amplitude of pure knowledge resplendent with merits developed through my association with you all, I now merge in the Supreme Brahman. (*sloka* 100)

Part II

yoga and western psychology

5

Freud, Jung, and Yoga on Memory

Modern Western psychology has rejected Yoga as a valid form of psychology. Yoga is dismissed as yet another version of Eastern metaphysics and mysticism. But there is one promising point of contact between Yoga and modern psychology, namely, an apparent parallel between the modern psychology of memory and the Yoga notion of *karma*. This is especially notable if a comparison is made of the conception of *karma* found in Patañjali's *Yoga Sūtras*[1] and the views of the contemporary psychologists Sigmund Freud[2] and Carl Jung.[3] For both the ancient Yoga of Patañjali and the modern psychology of Freud and Jung, memory, motivation, and the unconscious are intimately intertwined.

Karma is described by Patañjali as a memory trace recorded in the unconscious by any action or thought a person has done. The Westerner should especially note that for Yoga a thought is as real as an action; in fact, in the Yoga view, we think first and then act, and thought is of psychological importance. The karmic memory trace (*saṁskāra*) remains in the unconscious as a predisposition towards doing the same action or thought again in the future. All that is required is that the appropriate set of circumstances present themselves, and the karmic memory trace, like a seed that has been watered and given warmth, bursts forth as an impulsion toward the same kind of action or thought from which it originated. If, through the exercise of free choice, one chooses to act on the impulse and do the same action or thought again, then that karmic seed is allowed to flower, resulting in a reinforcing of the memory trace within the unconscious. Sufficient repetitions of the same action or thought produce a strengthening of the predisposition (*saṁskāra*), and the establishing of a "habit pattern" or *vāsanā*. Such a karmic habit pattern or *vāsanā* can be taken as the Yoga equivalent for the modern psychological notion of motivation.[4] The unconscious, in Yoga terminology, is nothing more than the sum total of all stored-up karmic traces from the thoughts and actions done in this and previous lives.

Many similarities with the ancient Yoga of Patañjali are found when the development of recent thinking regarding memory, motivation, and the unconscious is reviewed. Modern psychological theory seems to take its rise from two quite opposing philosophic conceptions of the human mind. According to John Locke, the mind is essentially passive in nature, while in the view of Gottfried Wilhelm Leibniz, its nature is active.[5] Locke assumed the mind of the individual to be a *tabula rasa*, or blank wax tablet, at birth and to acquire content passively through the impact of sensation and the interaction or association of traces left behind by such stimuli. This Lockean view of mental activity as a result of traces upon the "wax tablet" of the mind is similar to the Yoga understanding of *saṁskāras*, or memory traces, left within the *citta* (mind) by previous actions or thoughts. Robert Woodworth, the dean of American psychology in the 1920s and 1930s, noted that the stimulus-response traces, although originally activated by motivating stimuli external to them, may presently, after continued activation, become a drive.[6] In this way Woodworth extends the simple memory stimulus-mechanism of Locke's psychology so that motivation or drive is also accounted for, just as in Yoga the *saṁskāra* is not merely a memory trace but also an impulse toward further action.

The Lockean viewpoint, which has dominated most British and American psychology, has, in addition to the above similarity, a basic difference with Patañjali's Yoga. Whereas for the Lockean psychologists, each newborn child begins life with an empty mind, a *tabula rasa*, as it were. Yoga psychology emphasizes that at birth the mind (*citta*) carries with it a storehouse of *vāsanās*, or habit patterns, built up over a beginningless series of previous lives. While Woodworth's notions of memory and drive seem restricted to the personal experience of one lifetime, Patañjali's Yoga accounts for memory and motivation in terms of this and all previous lives. The difficulty which Locke, Woodworth, and their followers encounter in this regard, which is not a problem in Yoga, is the question of how to account for the many drives, or instinctual patterns of behavior, which the newborn child evidences immediately at birth and before any learning has taken place.

The Leibnizian approach in modern psychology, with its assumption that the mind is genetically active rather than passive, seems to avoid this last-mentioned difficulty, and in some ways is closer to the Yoga notion of *vāsanās*. Much of the dynamic psychology which has characterized European thinking (for example, Brentano, Freud, and the Gestalt theorists) is based on the assumptions of Leibniz. For Leibniz, a child begins life not as a passive wax tablet, but as a consciousness composed of inherent seed ideas which actively structure incoming stimuli and in so doing achieve greater actualization and motive force. Thus for Leibniz, as for Yoga psychology, there are degrees of consciousness, since the ideas grow from *petites perceptions*, which are to some degree unconscious, into their full flowering or actualization in conscious awareness.[7] Implicit in the thought of Leibniz, therefore, are the notions of inherent psychological structures and their resulting drives as well as various degrees of conscious awareness. As we shall see, much of this thinking is carried over into the psychological theories of Freud and Jung. Although the Leibnizian tradition in modern psychology seems, on balance, to have a good deal in common with the Yoga notion of *karma*, there is one aspect of Yoga that is quite out of step with Leibniz, that is, the Yoga notion of the *puruṣa*, or self as an individual pure consciousness, unchanging and eternal, which shines forth undimmed once all obstructing *karma* has been removed. Such a notion of the self seems totally foreign to modern psychology, whether it be of a Lockean or Leibnizian cast. But if the karmic processes of Yoga prior to the realization of *kaivalya* (final release of the *puruṣa*, or self, from its apparent entrapment in the *karma* of *prakṛti*) are taken as the point of focus, then it appears that there is much in common between the Leibnizian tradition within modern psychology and Patañjali's Yoga.

FREUD AND *KARMA*

Neurophysiological psychologists, such as Karl Pribram, have moved away from the simple (Lockean) spinal reflex model of memory to a Freudian (Leibnizian) theory which combines memory and motivation in a way very similar to the Yoga notions of *karma*. In his article "The Foundation of Psychoanalytic Theory: Freud's Neuropsychological Model,"[8] Karl Pribram takes us back to a little-known aspect of Freud's thought, namely, Freud's "Scientific Project," containing the view that at the neurophysiological level motive and memory are intimately intertwined.[9] The problem which Freud poses is exactly the one which the Yoga notion of karmic memory traces, or *saṁskāras*, seeks to answer. Freud asks the question: how can an organism remain sensitive to new excitations, yet at the same time develop the stabilities necessary to retain traces of prior stimulation? On the philosophical level, it is the problem of freedom and determinism. In relation to *karma*, it is the paradox that, although *karma* predisposes one to act or think in a particular way, still freedom of choice is said to be retained.[10] From the perspective of modern neurophysiological psychology, Pribram puts the problem this way: if the receptive aspects of a neural network are emphasized, "then the behaviour of the net is continually modified—i.e., the net is stimulus bound—and it retains little. If, on the other hand, the retentive capacities of the network are overemphasized, 'one-trial learning' and inability to allow subsequent modification characterizes the behaviour of the system."[11]

In addressing this problem, Freud abandons the view that sensory and memory mechanisms are neurologically separable and adopts the idea, which has become popular in neurophysiology, that receptor excitation repeatedly transmitted through the nervous system lowers synaptic resistance. "Memory is, according to this notion, a grooving or *bahnung* of transmission pathways in the nervous system."[12] Sir John Eccles, in his review of research findings, supports such a theory of memory and identifies the probable neurophysiological processes involved.

> It is attractive to conjecture that with memories enduring for years, there is some structural basis in the way of changed connectivities in the neuronal machinery. This would explain that there is a tendency for the replay of the spatiotemporal patterns of neural activity that occurred in the initial experience. This replaying in the brain would be accompanied by remembering in the mind. . . . The neurobiological level of memory is illustrated by a study of synaptic structure and synaptic action under conditions either of enhanced activity or of disuse. In this way it is shown that there are modifiable synapses that could be responsible for memory because they are greatly enhanced by activity and depleted by disuse. . .[13]

In terms of the actual neurological processes involved, Eccles concludes on the basis of experiments that there is good evidence that the spine synapses on the dendrites of neurons in the cerebral cortex and the hippocampus are modifiable to a high degree and exhibit a prolonged potentiation that could be the physiological expression of the memory process.[14] It is suggested that increased potentiation could result from either growth (hypertrophy) of the dendritic spine synapses or branching of the spines to form secondary spine synapses. By contrast, disuse is seen to result in a regression and depletion of spine synapses (Figure 1). That this psychobiological approach to memory is still very current and can be seen in a recent article by Francis Crick and Christof Koch.[15] Their focus is still on possible memory mechanisms located at the synapse, although the thinking as to what may be happening is somewhat more sophisticated regarding short- and long-term memory. Yet, the Freud-Eccles-Pribram approach discussed here is still a viable possibility.

The above theorizing by Freud and experimentation by Eccles may well serve as the modern explanation of the physiological character of *karmic saṁskāras* and *vāsanās*, an explanation which in Patañjali's time involved a long and detailed discussion as to how the *guṇas*, or constituents of consciousness (*sattva*, *rajas*, and *tamas*), function in the various karmic states.[17] In ancient Yoga terminology, the structuring of a memory trace was described as an accumulation of a latent deposit of *karma*, which would have as its neural basis a significant *tamas*, or physical structure component, perhaps parallel to enlarged dendritic spines of modern physiology. The Yogic notion of habit patterns, or *vāsanās*, as resulting from repetitions of a particular memory trace, or *saṁskāra*, fits well with the modern idea of growth at the synaptic spines.

The Yoga notion that the repetition of a particular *saṁskāra* results in a habit pattern, or *vāsanā*, assumes that memory and motivation are two aspects of the same psychological process. Freud, too, called attention to the intimate linkage of motive and memory. Motivation in Freud's view is selection, and selection is to a large degree the result of memory traces of prior experience.[18] Freud's analysis of the neurophysiological process required is as follows. Every neuron must be presumed to have several paths of connections with other neurons. Consequently, the possibility exists for choice among various neural pathways. But, as the Yoga theory of *karma* points out, people do not behave as if all paths are equally likely. Therefore, particular motivational patterns must be provided for in the functioning of the neural network. Freud

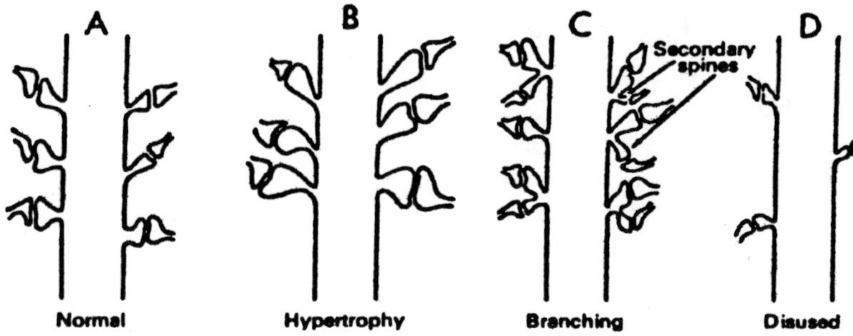

Figure 1. The drawings are designed to convey the changes in spine synapses that are postulated to occur with growth in B and C and with regression in D.[16]

accomplished this in terms of "cathexis," or the buildup, through repetition, of neural energy at a particular synaptic spine, which leads to transmitted excitation only under the conditions appropriate to that neural network. Thus, on the same neuron there could exist several synaptic spines each connected to different neural networks. Choice occurs when, as the impulse reaches the neuron, one of the several possible neural networks is selected. In Freud's view, the selection procedure prevents purely random transmission and operates on the basis of the cathexis, or potential energy buildup, at each synaptic spine.[19] This would be the neurophysiological correlate for the motivational, or *karmic*, predisposition in psychic functioning.

As Pribram makes clear, Freud in his "Project" did not succeed in solving "the question of how neural impulses are directed through a net, and under what conditions such selective direction leads to an adapted repetition of the neuronal pattern."[20] But in posing this important problem, says Pribram, Freud was far ahead of his time. Only recently has neurophysiology attained the laboratory techniques to study simultaneously what goes on in different portions of a neuron. In theory, both Yoga and Freud agree that memory and motivation are parts of a single psychic process which also embodies choice or selection. It would seem that only now has the science of neurophysiology advanced to the point where this theory can be empirically tested. Perhaps the experimental evidence, when obtained, will help to clarify the paradox which still remains, namely, to what degree is this choice or selection process free or determined?

In addition to his "Scientific Project," which he seems to have given up around 1895, Freud dealt with memory and motivation in the development of his theory of psychoanalysis. There, Freud argues that when our sense organs are stimulated, mental pictures are created of the perceived objects and preserved as memory traces in the unconscious.[21] These memory traces become associated with motivation when the personality becomes engaged in the process of tension reduction, as, for example, when a baby becomes hungry, triggering memories of the sight, smell, taste, and feel of food. This process, which produces a memory image of an object that is needed to reduce a tension, Freud called a primary process.[22] When such processes are perceived as threatening (e.g., in certain cases of sexual desire), they may be repressed so as to defend the person from dangerous desires (e.g., sexual desire that could lead to incest) or from traumatic experiences. Thus a whole series of associated memories may be repressed from conscious experience but continue to exist in the unconscious.[23] While Yoga psychology does not explicitly deal with Freud's insight regarding the defense mechanism of repression, both agree that memories are created at the conscious level, are stored in the unconscious, and have motivational power. As noted above, for both Freud and Yoga, the bulk of the psychic memory/motivation processes is within the unconscious. Freud, following the Leibnizian notion of *petites perceptions* growing into full-flowered conscious actualizations, taught that most of the motivation we experience in everyday life comes from the unconscious. In Freud's view, the forgetting of names, erroneously carried out actions, chance, and superstition are all accountable in terms of memories and motivations within the unconscious.[24] Yoga, with its conception of the unconscious as a huge storehouse of karmic seeds (*bījas*) constantly seeking to sprout forth into conscious actualization, would seem to be largely in agreement. But whereas Yoga assumes that at the conscious level there is a real possibility for the operation of free choice in either negating the karmic impulse or allowing it to actualize fully, Freud seems convinced that there is no such thing as free will. Of course, Freud allows that at the level of conscious awareness one feels sure that he could just as easily have acted differently, that he acted of his own free will and without any motives. But, says Freud, a careful psychoanalysis reveals that such so-called "free actions" for which no conscious motive can be identified are under the control of the unconscious. "What is thus left free from the one side receives its motive from the other side, from the unconscious, and determinism in the psychic realm is thus carried out uninterruptedly."[25] It is with this final stand in favour of the absolute determinism of the unconscious that Freud sharply diverges from Yoga. In Freud's view, the most that the conscious processes can hope to achieve is the ability to deal with the unconscious in a rational and insightful way. While the *Yoga Sūtras* agree with Freud that the pain and frustrations one experiences are caused by the *kleśas*, or drives of the unconscious,[26] Yoga clearly goes beyond the Freudian counsel that one must learn to live intelligently with such tension and discomfort. For Patañjali the goal of Yoga is the complete overcoming of the karmic traces and thus, in the end, the annihilation of the unconscious.[27] As we shall see, the approach of Carl Jung attempts to chart a middle course between these two extremes.

JUNG AND KARMA

The psychology of Carl Jung evidences both the thinking of his Western teacher, Sigmund Freud, and the influence of Patañjali's *Yoga Sūtras*.[28] A few years after his break with Freud, Jung turned to India and the East to obtain support for his differing views.[29] Although Jung remains resolutely Western and, along with Freud, denies that the unconscious could ever be totally overcome or destroyed, Jung is influenced by the Yoga notion of *karma* in important ways.[30] Jung seeks out a middle course between the determinism of Freud and the *Yoga Sūtra* ideal of absolute freedom once all *karma* is annihilated, or "burnt up," to use the Yoga metaphor. Jung, like Freud, simply cannot conceive of the unconscious ever becoming completely known. In a letter to W. Y. Evans-Wentz, Jung makes his position clear: "You can expand your consciousness so that you even cover a field that had been unconscious to you before . . . and there is absolutely no reason to believe then that there is not a million times more unconscious material beyond that little bit of new acquisition."[31] But in opposition to Freudian determinism and in line with Yoga, Jung gives considerable weight to the creative activity of the individual's ego-consciousness. This is seen in the multitude of different and unique ways that the common content of the collective unconscious is individuated and made present in the awareness of each of us. In Jung's thought, such individuation is genuinely creative and is to that extent an expression of freedom, but the essential content provided the individuation process by the collective unconscious and the external environment is *a priori* a given and therefore a necessity against which the freedom of the creative process is constrained. Jung's psychological process by which the innate contents of the unconscious are creatively individuated into conscious awareness within each psyche is therefore an attempt at a middle way between the extremes of freedom and determinism.

Just as in Yoga theory the contents of the unconscious are described as memory traces (*saṁskāras*), so also Jung conceives of the unconscious as containing the psychobiological memory of our ancestral past. The way we ordinarily think of memory, as, for example, when we memorize something for an examination, is called by Jung "an artificial acquisition consisting mostly of printed paper."[32] Here Jung is referring to our usual functioning at the level of consciousness only. At the conscious level, if we are asked to learn something of our past, we go to a history book and "memorize" it. For Jung, this is not real memory but merely an artificial acquisition. Real memory involves raising to consciousness the ancestral traces or archetypes which, in Jung's view, are inherent in the collective unconscious of each human being.

Although Jung did not ground his thinking on neurophysiology of the sort proposed by Freud, Jung did produce a detailed theory of the unconscious. Jung divided the contents of the unconscious into two kinds. The first, the contents of the collective unconscious, Jung suggested, are composed of the psychic heritage or history passed on to us by our animal ancestors, primitive human ancestors, ethnic group, nation, tribe, and family.[33] Although these collective memories determine our psychic life to a high degree, Jung described them as being "neutral" and becoming filled with content only when they come into contact with consciousness. As Gerhard Adler notes,

> In his later writings Jung expanded and developed the concept of the archetype considerably. He distinguished sharply between the irrepresentable, transcendental archetype *per se* and its visible manifestation in consciousness as the archetypal image or symbol. Moreover the archetype *per se* appears to be an *a priori* conditioning factor in the human psyche, comparable to the biological "pattern of behaviour," a "disposition" which starts functioning at a given moment in the development of the human mind and arranges the material of consciousness into definite patterns.[34]

Jung admitted that direct evidence for these inherited memory complexes was not available, but he argued that psychic manifestations such as the complexes, images, and symbols that we encounter in dreams, fantasies, and visions are indirect empirical evidence.[35] The second kind of content found in the unconscious consists of past experiences of the individual's own lifetime that have been either forgotten or repressed. These Jung calls the memories of the personal unconscious.[36] Empirical evidence for their existence is demonstrated when they can be recalled during hypnosis or certain drug states and yet remain unknowable during ordinary consciousness. It is the making present of these two types of psychic contents from the unconscious that Jung views as real memory, as opposed to the artificial memory of something memorized from a book. We examine Jung's account of the psychological processes involved in memory in more detail in chapter 6.

In Yoga, the unconscious is nothing more than the stored up *saṁskāras* left behind as memory traces of past thoughts or actions. Like the forgotten or repressed contents of Jung's personal unconscious, some of the *saṁskāras* will be the memory traces of thoughts or actions undertaken during this lifetime. But where Yoga differs from Jung is that the vast majority of the *saṁskāras* making up the unconscious come not from the collective history of mankind but rather from the individual history of that particular person's past lives. For Yoga, the vast majority of the *saṁskāras* stored in the unconscious are not the forgotten materials from this life, but memory traces from the actions and thoughts in the innumerable past lives of the individual. Whereas Jung is willing to give sympathetic consideration to this notion of *saṁskāras* from the past, if it is understood as a kind of collective psychic heredity, he flatly rejects the idea of reincarnation of the individual soul. For Jung, "there is no inheritance of individual prenatal or pre-uterine memories, but there are undoubtedly inherited archetypes."[37] These archetypes are "the universal dispositions of the mind, and they are to be understood as analogous to Plato's forms (*eidola*), in accordance with which the mind organizes its contents."[38]

The other major difference between Jung and Yoga has to do with their differing assessments as to the degree to which the memory and unconscious can be known. For Yoga, meditation is a psychological process whereby the *saṁskāras*, or memory traces, of past actions or thoughts are purged from the "storehouse" of the unconscious. As these memories of the past are brought up from the unconscious, their contents momentarily pass through our conscious awareness. It is in this way, says Yoga, that we come to know all forgotten actions and thoughts from this life as well as all actions and thoughts composing our past lives. Thus the claim of the great *yogins*, such as Gautama Buddha, that through intense meditation all *saṁskāras* are brought up to the level of awareness, and exhaustive knowledge of one's past lives is achieved. This yogic accomplishment not only does away with memory, since everything is now present knowledge, but also with the unconscious, since it was nothing but the sum total of the *saṁskāras*, or memory traces of the past. A perfected yogin, such as the Buddha, therefore, is said to be totally present—a mind uncluttered by the *saṁskāras* of an unconscious psyche. As the Zen master Eido Roshi put it, meditation is the removal of mental defilements. Yoga is like a mental vacuum cleaner that removes from our minds all the *saṁskāras* collected during this and previous lives.[39] Patañjali defines yoga as the removal or destruction of all *karmic saṁskāras* from previous lives until a completely clear and discriminating mind is achieved.[40] For Patañjali's Yoga, *saṁskāras* or memory traces function as obstacles to true knowledge of reality, and their removal by yogic meditation results in omniscience.[41]

Jung saw that the Yoga viewpoint led to a dissolution of ego and individuality, and thus to a completely different conception of freedom. Freedom, to Jung, implied the creative activity of each person's ego in individuating the archetypes. This Jungian "individual freedom" is the polar opposite of the Yoga teaching that true freedom is known only when one gives up all ego-activity. Jung could agree that Yoga for the Easterner, or "individuation" for the Westerner, would help an individual to recover knowledge of thoughts or actions of this life which had been forgotten or repressed. He would also allow that the same techniques could put one in touch with the archetypes, or psychic heredity, of the collective unconscious. But here Jung's theory diverges from Patañjali's Yoga in three ways. The first difference is that, for Jung, one cannot speak in terms of individual *saṁskāras* of previous lives but only of collective predispositions (archetypes) passed on by a person's ancestors. A second difference is that whereas for Yoga the *saṁskāras* are obstructions which must be removed for the achievement of knowledge, for Jung it is through the shaping of the materials of consciousness by the archetypal "memories" that knowledge of reality results. For Yoga, however, knowledge of reality is a given inherently present in the consciousness of each individual and requiring only the removal of obstructing and distorting memory traces (*saṁskāras*) for its full and complete revelation. In Jung's view, such a claim is one-sidedly subjective. It does not take seriously the experiential fact that the subjective categories of the mind do not possess knowledge themselves, but merely shape external stimuli so that perceptual knowledge results. The one-sided Yoga theory, therefore, is to be dismissed as unwarranted metaphysical speculation.[42]

A third difference arises directly from the different value given memory by the two approaches, and from the Yoga claim that all *saṁskāras*, all memory, can be removed. Jung agrees with the Yoga contention that ego, or "I-ness," results from the continuity of memory.[43] But Jung flatly rejects the Yoga notion that since the ego-sense that memories produce is composed of nothing but obstructing *saṁskāras*, true knowledge requires that ego-sense be removed. Thus with regard to the Yoga claims of realizing egolessness, Jung concludes that such a state is both a philosophical and a psychological impossibility. The Yoga claim of omniscience must also be rejected, for there will always be more of the unconscious to be explored.

This chapter has examined points of contact between the understanding of *karma* as set forth in Patañjali's *Yoga Sūtras* and the modern theorizing of Freud and Jung with regard to memory, motivation, and the unconscious. Freud's thinking, following the Leibnitzian tradition with its assumption that the mind is genetically active rather than passive, seems parallel to the yogic notion of *vāsanās*, or karmic drives, within the unconscious. In his little-known *Project for a Scientific Psychology*, Freud attempted a neurophysiological solution to the question: how can an organism remain sensitive to new excitations yet at the same time retain traces of prior stimulation—the very problem which the Yoga notion of karmic memory traces, or *saṁskāras*, seeks to answer. More philosophically stated, it is the paradox that although *karma* predisposes one to act or think in a particular way, still freedom of choice is said to be retained. Freud's neurophysiological theory provides for a kind of "grooving" of transmission pathways in the nervous system. The research of Sir John Eccles suggests that this "grooving" takes place by growth in the spines on neuron dendrites which facilitates synaptic transmission of the impulse along a particular neural network. This work of Freud and Eccles indicates that there are modifiable synapses that could be the modern neurophysiological explanation for karmic *saṁskāras* and *vāsanās*, an explanation which in Patañjali's day was attempted in terms of *guṇa* theory.

Although both Freud and Yoga theory agree that the bulk of the psychic memory processes are usually within the unconscious, there is disagreement as to the deterministic nature of such processes. In Freud's view, the choices offered between several neural networks on a single neuron are largely determined by motives which are operative at the unconscious level. Or, in terms of his psychoanalytic theory, Freud sees all memory from sensory experience or repressions existing as memory images within the unconscious. Yoga, by contrast, treats the karmic processes as predispositions of greater or lesser strength but which always require an act of free choosing at the level of conscious awareness for either actualization or negation. With regard to this balance between unconscious impulses and free choice, the psychology of Carl Jung seems more in tune with Patañjali's Yoga. Jung provides for motivation from the unconscious in the form of the archetypes, but allows for free choice in his requirement that the archetype be creatively developed by each individual within his own ego-consciousness. According to Jung, such individuation of the archetype is genuinely creative and is to that extent an expression of freedom. Although Jung's notion of the archetypes is similar to and may well have been influenced by Patañjali's theory of *saṁskāras*, three ways in which Jung differs from Yoga are identified: (1) In Jung's view, one cannot speak in terms of individual *saṁskāras* of previous lives, but only of collective predispositions or archetypes passed on by a person's ancestors. (2) Whereas for Yoga the *saṁskāras* are obstructions which must be removed for the realization of knowledge, for Jung it is through the shaping of the materials of consciousness by the archetypal "memories" that knowledge of reality results. (3) While Jung agrees with the Yoga contention that ego, or I-ness, results from the continuity of memory, he rejects the Yoga notion that, since the ego-sense that memories produce is composed of nothing but obstructing *saṁskāras*, true knowledge requires that ego-sense be transcended.

In conclusion, it may be said that the ancient Yoga conception of *karma* can be shown to have points of significant contact with modern psychology. Patañjali's Yoga has always viewed memory and motivation as aspects of the same psychological process, a position which has been adopted by contemporary Western cognitive psychologists.[44] Freud's emphasis upon the unconscious and his delineation of its likely neurophysiological basis provide a modern scientific basis for a good portion of Patañjali's *karma* theory, which theory on the other hand challenges the throughgoing unconscious determinism of the Freudian point of view. In attempting a middle path between freedom and determinism, Jung's psychology is seen to be more in line with Yoga. However, Jung's stress on the collective nature of the unconscious and its inability to be completely known is challenged by Patañjali's theory, which sees *karma* as individual and open to complete removal in the quest for omniscience.

6

Where Jung Draws the Line in His Acceptance of Patañjali's Yoga

In the formation of his psychological theory, Carl Jung was for a time strongly influenced by Patañjali's Yoga Psychology.[1] The period of influence was mainly in the 1920s, but by the end of the 1930s Jung's main attention turned back to Western thought.[2] This is especially evident if the cognitive aspects of his psychology, for example, the processes of memory, perception, and thinking are analyzed in relation to the corresponding concepts found in Patañjali's *Yoga Sūtras*. Such an analysis shows that at least one of the reasons Jung could not completely identify with Patañjali's Yoga was the lack of distinction between philosophy and psychology that seems to typify much Eastern thought. In line with other modern Western thinkers, Jung claimed to follow the scientific method of keeping a clear distinction between the description of cognitive processes, on the one hand, and truth claims attesting to the objective reality of such cognitions, on the other. Any reductionistic collapsing of philosophy into psychology or vice versa is the cause of what Jung critically calls Eastern intuition over-reaching itself. For Jung, this over-reaching of yoga is especially evident in the widespread Eastern notion that the individual ego can be completely transcended and some form of universal consciousness achieved.[3] In Jung's eyes, this was nothing more than the psychological projection of an idea which had no foundation in human experience.

Jung viewed the East as making such errors because it had not yet reached the high level of self-awareness achieved in the modern Western development of scientific thought. The Indian, says Jung, is still pre-Kantian. In India, therefore, "there is no psychology in our sense of the word. India is 'pre-psychological.'"[4] In a 1958 letter Jung wrote, "There is no psychology worthy of this name in East Asia, but instead a philosophy consisting entirely of what we would call psychology."[5] In Jung's view, Eastern psychology was nothing more than a kind of scholastic description of psychic processes with no necessary connection to empirical facts. Because of this lack of empirical method, said Jung, Eastern thought suffers "a curious detachment from the world of concrete particulars we call reality."[6] As evidence for this contention, Jung reported that Easterners, while gifted in seeing things in their totality, had great difficulty in perceiving the whole in terms of its empirical parts. For example, of his conversation with the Chinese scholar Hu Shih, Jung said, ". . . it was as though I had asked him to bring me a blade of grass, and each time he had dragged along a whole meadow for me. . . . Each time I had to extract the detail for him from an irreducible totality."[7] The East, said Jung, still views reality metaphysically in terms of the whole, and describes the whole in cognitive projections which often have little to do with the nominalistic concepts of the empiricist. In a 1955 letter to a theological student, Jung makes clear that whereas modern psychology (including Freud's Psychoanalysis and Jung's own Analytical Psychology) has an empirical foundation, the older psychologies of the East and the medieval West are founded on metaphysical concepts which often have little relation to empirical facts. It is clear that Jung views his own work as scientific while that of the older psychologies is of a quite different order—"opinion rather than fact."[8]

As a champion of modern scientific psychology, Jung was not unaware of its hazards. Because of its focus on the minutiae of empirical evidence, modern psychology often lost sight of the larger whole. Emphasis upon the holistic or collective nature of the unconscious was seen by Jung as one of his major contributions in helping to restore the balance between the part and the whole in modern Western thought. Jung's main empirical evidence in this regard was the dreams and drawings produced by himself and his patients. He appealed to the Eastern stress on the wholeness or collective nature of reality as providing not additional empirical evidence, but rather historical and literary parallels to his scientific discoveries.

It is evident in the above discussion that the underlying distinction which determines where Jung draws the line in his acceptance of Yoga comes from his holding firmly to modern Western scientific method.[9] The essential basis of the modern scientific approach is that it carefully avoids any reductionism between psychology and philosophy or any confusion between the two. One of the more general statements of the domain and method of modern psychology is offered by the philosopher Gilbert Ryle.[10] Ryle argues that psychology is that science which provides explanations for the kinds of behavior for which we can ordinarily give no explanation. Ryle offers the following examples: "I do not know why I was so tongue-tied in the presence of a certain acquaintance; why I dreamed a certain dream last night; why I suddenly saw in my mind's eye an uninteresting street corner of a town that I hardly know; why I chatter more rapidly after the air-raid siren is heard; or how I came to address a friend by the wrong Christian name."[11] In addition there are the cases of perceptual illusion such as why a straight line cutting through certain cross-hatchings looks bent, which we cannot explain from our own knowledge. Psychology has also devised its own particular methods for measuring both ordinary and unusual sorts of behavior. The hallmark of this method is that it is empirical in nature. Ryle effectively argues against "the false notion that psychology is the sole empirical study of people's mental powers, propensities, and performances, together with its implied false corollary that 'the mind' is what is properly describable only in the technical terms proprietary to psychological research."[12] To illustrate his argument, Ryle offers the analogy that England cannot be described solely in seismological terms. With this contention Jung would agree. But Jung's additional plea is that the psychological enterprise must be carried on with the larger perspective of the other empirical disciplines in view. A complete knowledge of England requires geographical, historical, botanical, and other studies, along with the seismological enterprise. Western empirical psychology must be aware of the scientific achievements of physiology, anthropology, physics, history, philosophy, religion, and so on. The difference between the East and the West is that although the East includes all of life in its domain of knowledge, it achieves this holistic view by an uncritical lumping together of all knowledge. This has had the result of confusion and reductionism between disciplines and, in Jung's view, is at least part of the reason for Eastern thought losing contact with reality and indulging in "cognitive projection" rather than empirical observation. Let us test out Jung's contention in this regard by comparing his analysis of memory, perception, and knowing with the descriptions found in the *Yoga Sūtras* of Patañjali.

MEMORY AND THE UNCONSCIOUS

The unique aspect of Jung's view of memory is that it functions at the level of the unconscious as well as at the level of the conscious psyche. Indeed for Jung, real memory necessarily first resides in the collective unconscious in a subliminal form. Only after such psychic contents are raised or individuated beyond a certain threshold level of psychic energy is consciousness of the memory achieved. For Jung's psychology, memory and other cognitive functions, such as perception, intuition, imagination, thinking, and feeling, all exist in subliminal form in the unconscious. The main difference between the occurrence of these functions in the unconscious as opposed to the conscious is that in the former they possess less psychic energy or intensity and thus remain below the threshold of awareness.[13]

As we saw in the previous chapter, Jung distinguishes our memorizing of information from notes for an examination—which he calls an "artificial acquisition"—from "real memory," which for him is the raising to conscious awareness of the ancestral traces contained in the archetypes of the collective unconscious inherent in each person. Real memory involves knowing ourselves from within rather than from books. Jung does allow that memories from experiences during one's own lifetime (that have been forgotten or repressed) make up the contents of what he calls the personal unconscious. For Patañjali's Yoga, as we outlined in chapter 5, both memories and the unconscious are accounted for in terms of *saṁskāras*, or memory traces of an individual's actions or thoughts in this or previous lives stored up in the unconscious. As we previously noted, Jung disagreed with the Yoga idea that memories of past lives could be individual and that the contents of the unconscious were these individual memories or *saṁskāras*. For Jung, to the extent that memories from past lives exist in the unconscious, they are collective rather than individual in nature. Jung called them the archetypes.

Also, as shown in chapter 5, Jung disagreed with Yoga over the degree to which memory and the unconscious can be known. While for Yoga, the goal of Yoga is the raising of all memory traces, or *saṁskāras*, from the unconscious to conscious awareness, Jung was convinced that such a goal was not realizable. Jung thought that no matter how much material is raised to the level of conscious awareness, there will always be more left in the unconscious. The Yoga claim that all the memory contents can, through the meditation techniques of Yoga, be made known, and thus cause the unconscious to cease to exist, is simply impossible in Jung's view. The parallel Yoga claim of omniscience resulting from the raising of all the memory contents to the conscious level (e.g., the Buddha's claim to knowledge of all past lives) is, for Jung, evidence of Yoga's lack of an empirical grounding.

Jung was well acquainted with these Yoga teachings of Patañjali. In his 1939 Summer Semester Lectures at the Eidgenössische Technische Hochschule, Zürich, Jung wrote his own commentary on the claims of the *Yoga Sūtras*.[14] Jung agreed that there were psychological techniques such as Yoga that would enable us to get to know the unconscious and at least some of its memory contents. While he allowed that Patañjali's yogic meditation may be an appropriate technique for the Easterner, Jung argued that his process of active imagination was more suitable for the Westerner.[15] Jung's reasoning here was that a rigorously disciplined yogic practice such as Patañjali's would only aggravate the already chronic Western ailment, namely, overdevelopment of the will and the conscious control of the psyche. Jung felt that the better way for Western person to overcome his or her encapsulation within the conscious level and get to know the contents of the unconscious was through the process of fantasizing or active imagination—a technique which Jung had developed in his own psychological practice.[16]

Aside from this difference as to the best technique to use in getting to know and control the unconscious, Jung saw that the Yoga viewpoint led to a complete dissolution of ego and individuality, and this he felt to be nothing more than fanciful speculation. Jung could agree that Yoga, for the Easterner, or active imagination, for the Westerner, would help an individual to recover knowledge of thoughts or actions of this life which had been forgotten or repressed. He would also allow that the same technique could put one in touch with the archetypes or psychic heredity of the collective unconscious.

Jung agrees with the Yoga contention that ego, or 'I-ness', results from the continuity of memory.[17] But Jung flatly rejects the Yoga notion that since the ego-sense that memories produce is composed of nothing but obstructing *saṁskāras*, true knowledge requires that ego-sense be removed. In a 1939 letter to W. Y. Evans-Wentz, Jung speaks strongly against the notion of 'egoless knowing' prevalent in both Hindu and Buddhist yoga: "No matter how far an *ekstasis* [religious ecstasy] goes or how far consciousness can be extended, there is still the continuity of the apperceiving ego which is essential to all forms of consciousness. . . . Thus it is absolutely impossible to know what I would experience when that "I" which could experience didn't exist any more. . . ."[18]

Thus with regard to the Yoga claims of realizing egolessness, Jung concludes that such a state is both a philosophical and a psychological impossibility. The Yoga claim of omniscience must also be rejected, for there will always be more of the unconscious to be explored. "Agnosticism," says Jung, "is my duty as a scientist."[19]

PERCEPTION

The idea of an egoless state of consciousness has had a considerable influence on the Yoga view of perception. Patañjali taught that on the removal of the ego-producing and obstructing *saṁskāras*, a supernormal level of perception (*pratibhā*) is experienced.[20] *Pratibhā* or intuition is held to give noumenal knowledge of the object upon which the yogi is meditating. For Yoga, the ordinary psychic state which is dominated by ego-consciousness produces only everyday phenomenal knowledge of the object. For Patañjali, therefore, and for most Hindu and Buddhist schools of thought, there are two levels of perception.[21] On the lower level, the ego and its *saṁskāras* so obstruct the perception that only a distorted view of the whole object is seen. According to Patañjali's analysis, the distortion occurs when the perception of the object is mixed together in consciousness with the word we use in language to name the object and the meaning or idea which this name evokes. It is the perception of the object itself which is the true perception. The perceptions of the word-label and word-meaning are legacies of convention or past usage and as such are distorting *saṁskāras*. Once these two distorting memories are purged from consciousness so that the direct experience of the object alone remains, *pratibhā*, or the higher level of perception, has been achieved.[22] The yoga description of *pratibhā* perception suggests a consciousness so purged of all filtering or distorting *saṁskāras* that the object shines through it as through a perfectly pure pane of glass. It is as if the cognizing consciousness becomes completely devoid of its own nature and takes on the nature of the object itself.[23] The object in all its aspects and qualities stands fully revealed as in a single flash.[24] Jung's critique of this concept of *pratibhā*, or higher perception, is based upon his philosophic presupposition that it is impossible to have a knowing experience without the presence of a knower in consciousness. In the Yoga example of consciousness taking on the nature of the object, Jung argues, "There must always be somebody or something left over to experience the realization, to say, 'I know at-one-ment, I know there is no distinction.'"[25] It is simply impossible to completely dispense with the knowing ego.

> Even when I say "I know myself," an infinitesimal ego—the knowing "I"—is still distinct from "myself." In this as it were atomic ego, which is completely ignored by the essentially non-dualistic standpoint of the East, there nevertheless lies hidden the whole unabolished pluralistic universe and its unconquered reality. The experience of "at-one-ment" is one example of those "quick-knowing" realizations of the East, an intuition of what it would be like if one could exist and not exist at the same time.[26]

Jung's judgment as to what is really happening when the yogis think they are in a *pratibhā* state is found in his 1934 letter to the physicist Wolfgang Pauli. After suggesting that if you look long enough into a dark hole you perceive what is looking in, Jung argues that something like this is happening to the yogis. After looking long enough at the object, or at nothing, as in many yogic practices, the yogi becomes aware of his own psyche. Yoga, says Jung, is simply a special technique for introspection.[27]

Jung's own analysis of perception also results in what seems to be a two-level theory. There are the sense perceptions of ordinary experience at the conscious level, and then there is what Jung calls the process of intuition, which occurs mostly at the unconscious level. Whereas in Yoga one goes from ordinary sense experience to the higher level of *pratibhā*, or supersensuous perception, Jung starts with ordinary sense experience and then goes inward to the lower level of the unconscious.[28]

Ordinary sense perceptions, says Jung, are a result of the stimuli that stream into us from the outside world. We see, hear, taste, smell, and touch the world, and so we are conscious of it. The bare sense perceptions simply tell us that something is, but not what it is. To know what something is, says Jung, involves the more complicated analysis and evaluation of the sense perception by the cognitive processes of thinking and feeling. This second-order analysis of the bare sense perceptions Jung calls apperception.[29] For example, we hear a noise which, on analysis, strikes us as peculiar—an evaluation supplied by the feeling function—and is recognized as the noise that air-bubbles make when rising in the pipes of the heating system—an explanation provided by the thinking process.

Jung describes intuition as one of the basic functions of the psyche. He defines intuition as "perception of the possibilities inherent in a situation,"[30] sometimes called a "hunch." Whereas sense perception derives a conscious apprehension of reality, or things as they are, intuition derives an unconscious or inner conception of the potentialities of things. In viewing a mountain landscape, for example, the person who functions mainly at the level of sense perceptions will note every detail: the flowers, the colors of the rocks, the trees, and the waterfall, while the intuitive type will simply register the general atmosphere and color.[31] There are those situations encountered in life where everything appears quite normal at the level of conscious sense perceptions, yet the small inner voice of intuition tells us to "look out," for things are not as they should be. In such instances, suggests Jung, we have many subliminal perceptions, and from these, at the unconscious level, our hunches arise. This is perception by way of the unconscious.[32] Jung says that the wisdom intuition offers us, especially when we find ourselves thrust into primitive situations, comes from the archetypes, or memory traces, of the unconscious. While the archetypes of the collective unconscious make available to us in outline form the ways our ancestors have reacted in key situations, it is the function of intuition to bring this wisdom forward to the level of consciousness and to make it relevant by shaping and interpreting the sense impressions received from the external environment. It is the function of the ego to receive such creations of the intuitive process once the level of consciousness is reached.[33]

In contrast to the Yoga view of the highest level of consciousness as *pratibhā* or unlimited omniscience, Jung sees consciousness as a world full of restrictions.

> No consciousness can harbor more than a very small number of simultaneous perceptions. All else must be in shadow, withdrawn from sight. Any increase in the simultaneous contents immediately produces a dimming of consciousness, if not confusion to the point of disorientation. Consciousness not only requires, but is of its very nature strictly limited to, the few and hence the distinct.[34]

What the yogi imagines himself to be perceiving in the state of *pratibhā* would include the simultaneous sum total of all available sense perceptions plus all the subliminal contents of the unconscious. Jung calls this Eastern claim "a most audacious fantasy" and argues that the very maximum consciousness can achieve is to single out for perception a small part of the external sensory input and the vast store of subliminal psychic potentials in the unconscious. In Zen meditation, says Jung, what happens is that consciousness is emptied as far as possible of its perceived contents, which then "fall back" into the unconscious. The contents that "break through" into consciousness as the *satori*, or enlightenment, experience are far from random. They represent the natural healing and integrating tendency inherent in the archetypes of the collective unconscious. The allowing of new contents to come forward and be integrated at the level of the conscious ego is the Zen parallel to the therapeutic function of modern Western psychological techniques, such as Jung's notion of active imagination. In Jung's view, it is the unconscious and its contents that are Zen's "original man."[35]

Yet another perspective on Jung's understanding of perception is found in an explanation he writes to A. M. Hubbard regarding Hubbard's experiments with the psychedeletic drug mescaline. Jung describes the action of mescaline as paralyzing the normal selective and integrative functions of apperception. The bare sense perceptions are added to by the myriad of emotions, associations, and meanings that the sense perceptions evoke from the vast store of subliminal possibilities contained in the unconscious psyche. Jung writes, "These additions, if unchecked, would dissolve into or cover up the objective image by an infinite variety, a real 'fantasia' or symphony of shades and nuances both of qualities as well as of meanings."[36] Unlike the normal process of cognition where the ego and its apperceptive processes produce a "correct" representation of the object by excluding inappropriate subliminal perceptional variants, the anaesthetic action of mescaline upon the ego-consciousness opens the door to the riotous world of the unconscious. In Jung's view, it is better that this doorway to the unconscious be opened by the technique of active imagination, which leaves the integrative processes of the ego-consciousness functional, and thereby enables therapeutic gains to be made.[37]

The concept of intuitive perception is used by Jung to account for cases of extrasensory perception (ESP). ESP is simply seen as perception by way of the unconscious, and therefore should be thought of as a special case of intuition. In a 1945 letter, Jung says that he is entirely convinced of the existence of ESP and has left a place for ESP in his definition of intuition. What is needed now, he contends, is that physiology should follow his lead and leave room for paraphysiology.[38]

KNOWLEDGE

All Eastern schools of philosophy that adopt a two-level theory of perception also maintain that there are two levels of knowledge. Lower knowledge results when the sense organs come into contact with some object. This knowledge is limited by the factors of time, because the object is known in the present but not in the past or future; space because the object is known in the present location but not in other locations; by the efficiency of the sense organ; and by the distortions imposed by *saṁskāras* of past usage of word-label and meaning which attach themselves to the direct perception of the object. Because of these limitations, it is referred to as lower knowledge and is thought to be quite useful in everyday practical affairs but of little use if one is searching for true or absolute knowledge of the object.[39] Such higher knowledge can be realized only through the special yogic *pratibhā*, or supersensuous intuition of the object. The Sanskrit word *pratibhā*, which literally means a flash of light, is suggestive of the kind of cognition involved. Patañjali describes it as immediate and intensely clear. It is free from time and space limitations and from the distorting *saṁskāras* of word-labels, previously ascribed discursive meanings and ego-consciousness. It relies on neither the sense organs nor the rational intellect. The Sanskrit word most commonly employed in Eastern thought to refer to this higher knowledge is *prajñā*.[40]

Although *prajñā* is mentioned several times by Patañjali, it is perhaps best defined in *Yoga Sūtras* I: 47 and 48. *Prajñā* is knowledge of the truth, the essence. In it there is not even a trace of false knowledge.[41] Through the constant training of yoga, the mind is gradually freed from the distorting effects of conceptual thinking and from the *saṁskāras*, or memory traces, of the past. Finally the mind (*citta*) becomes so pure (*sattva*) that it merges with any object which may be presented to it. "No matter what this object may be, it is then fully illumined and its real nature perfectly brought out."[42]

While Eastern scholars claim that the above description of *prajñā* is based directly on the actual experiences of yogis and is therefore empirical evidence, Jung argues that it is nothing more than a fanciful projection. If the cognitive structures of ego-consciousness, conceptual thinking, and sense perception are not functioning in *prajñā*, as the yogis claim, then the trance they achieve can be nothing more than unconsciousness. If the yogi is unconscious, he can hardly be realizing absolute knowledge of the object. One cannot be fully aware and unconscious at the same time. For Jung this internal contradiction within Eastern thought is totally unacceptable.[43] The fact that this conflict does not seem to trouble Eastern scholars leads him to conclude that the Eastern intellect is underdeveloped when compared with the Western intellect.[44]

Jung's theory of knowledge also seems to have two levels. The lower level results from the ordinary reception of sense perceptions and the apperception of these in a routine mechanical fashion, almost totally without reference to the unconscious realm. The analysis of artificial memory, cited above, is a good example of what Jung means here. Although this may provide useful technical knowledge, it leaves a person cut off from his or her intuitive processes and from the deeper wisdom of the ages. Higher knowledge results when the intuitive processes engage the external sense perceptions with the *a priori* forms of the archetypes, so that a newly created and truly meaningful symbol is given birth in consciousness.[45] This is Jung's process of individuation, by which the ego through the cognitive processes of sensing, intuiting, thinking, and feeling employs the formal structures of the archetypes to appropriate selected sense apperceptions from the multitude of environmental stimuli. In this way both the inner archetypes and the external environment becomes known. As this integration of archetypes with external sense perceptions proceeds, a self is gradually individuated, or separated out, as the person's own particular uniqueness. For Jung the highest knowledge is knowledge of the self. This is achieved when the self becomes sufficiently integrated for the ego to recognize it as a unified whole.[46] It is through the integrating structure of the self, which extends outward from the ego in ever-expanding concentric circles, embracing both the conscious and the unconscious psyche, that the wisdom of the world is known. As Jung puts it, "Individuation does not shut one out from the world, but gathers the world to oneself."[47] For Jung it is the circular *maṇḍala* that best symbolizes the archetype of the self and helps to integrate the personality until the state of self-knowledge is finally realized. But regardless of how much we may integrate and make ourselves conscious through this process, "there will always exist an indeterminate and indeterminable amount of unconscious material which belongs to the totality of the self."[48] Given the necessity of the ego for conscious awareness, the limits of higher knowledge, for Jung, are much more restricted than the wide-open *prajñā* of the yogis. According to Jungian psychology, total knowledge of the self can never be achieved.

7

Mysticism in Jung and Patañjali's Yoga

MYSTICISM DEFINED

The study of mysticism has occupied an important place in almost all of the great religious traditions. In recent years, however, the term *mysticism* has been used so loosely in everyday language that its traditional meaning is in danger of becoming lost. Bookstores typically link mysticism with the occult and frequently display books on mysticism in the "occultism" section. Such psychic phenomena as visions, levitation, trances, and altered states of consciousness are frequently dubbed "mystical." Walter Principe reported the following newspaper item:

> Last May the *Toronto Star's* headline-writer announced: "Scientist offers electronic way to mysticism"—this to entice readers to an article about a "meditation machine" or revolving bed that is "intended," says the photo-caption, "to help people enjoy the spiritual experiences formerly available only to religious mystics."[1]

With such imprecision in the use of the term *mysticism* abounding, it is important that any scholarly discussion begin with a precise definition of the subject.

In his book entitled *Mysticism and Philosophy*, Walter Stace points out that the very word *mysticism* is an unfortunate one. "It suggests mist, and therefore foggy, confused, or vague thinking. It also suggests mystery and miraclemongering, and therefore hocus-pocus."[2] But when an examination is made of the experiences reported by the great mystics, something which is much different emerges. Rather than being "misty" or "confused," mystical experiences are typically described as clear illuminations having all the qualities of direct sensory perception. Stace, in fact, suggests that it is helpful to think of mystical experience as in some respects parallel to ordinary sense experience, that is, as a perception of a spiritual presence which is greater than humankind. Defining it as a perception, says Stace, allows one to avoid Russell's error of describing mysticism as only an emotion, and therefore as simply subjective.[3] The question raised is this: Does mystical experience, like sense experience, point to any objective reality, or is it a merely subjective psychological phenomenon? This question is, of course, one which is formulated by a philosopher for philosophical reasons, but it is a question which necessarily raises psychological issues. Is the psychological process of the mystical experience in some way analogous to sense perception? Or is it, as Rudolf Otto (following Immanuel Kant) suggests, something that begins amid all the sensory data of the natural world and indeed cannot exist without such data, and yet does not arise *out of* them but is merely occasioned by them.[4] Otto, of course, prefers an analogy to aesthetic experience as the best way of evoking a sense of the mystical. He also seems to suggest the existence of a separate psychological faculty specially suited for the reception of numinous stimuli emanating from the wholly other (the *numen*).

Frederick Copleston pointed out a paradox which is characteristic of mystical experience. "In the case of mysticism a man may be conscious of the fact that the experience described transcends the range of his own experience; and yet at the same time his reading and effort of understanding may be for him the occasion of a personal awareness of God."[5] On this point virtually all scholars agree. Mysticism is characterized by the experience of an unseen reality,[6] a spiritual presence,[7] a numen,[8] or an absolute[9] that is transcendent in that "it is identifiable neither with the empirical world as its appears to us in everyday experience and in natural science nor with the finite self considered as such . . ."[10] It is this very transcendent character of mystical experience that causes scholars to reject psychic phenomena, such as imaginative visions, voices, ecstasies, raptures, and so on, as not mystical in and of themselves. As Copleston puts it, "we all know that some people see things or hear voices without even a prima facie connection with the divine. And of course there are also pathological psychological states resembling ecstasy which can be accounted for by purely naturalistic explanations."[11] Mystical experience, by contrast, is transcendent of both the sensory experience of the empirical world and any all-encompassing identification with a finite ego of the sort which typifies pathological states.

Other than a general agreement that mystical experience is transcendent in nature and must not be confused with extraordinary psychic accomplishments and certain pathological states, there seems to be little consensus about the psychological processes involved. There is Stace's suggestion that something like sense perception is the process involved. Otto, however, rejects the perception analogy as too narrow; instead, in an analogy from aesthetics, he invokes a special mental faculty which would function amid the data of feeling, perception, and cognition, and yet somehow be independent of all of these. William James makes the very general suggestion that mystical experience of the transcendent occurs through the psychological processes of the subconscious self.[12] In the midst of this confusion and disagreement about the psychological processes involved, it is helpful to examine comparatively the thought of the Western psychologist Carl Jung and the Yoga psychologist Patañjali in relation to mystical experience.

MYSTICISM IN THE ANALYTICAL PSYCHOLOGY OF CARL JUNG

Writing his "Late Thoughts,"[13] Carl Jung puts down his own personal religious experience as clearly as may be found anywhere in his writings. There is no doubt that Jung's experience was highly mystical. All around himself Jung felt the forces of good and evil moving, but in the end the only thing that really mattered was the degree to which the individuated self could transcend these opposing forces.

It seems to have been Jung's view that as an isolated ego, a person would never succeed in reuniting the opposing forces. Those forces within the personality would simply overpower one's ego, and chaos would ensue. What saves us from this fate, said Jung, is the fact that deep within each of us is the God-image which is the psychological foundation of our psyche. The God-image, or archetype, is inherent in the collective unconscious as the primal stratum or foundational matrix. Jung's most significant religious experience did not focus on the reconciling of God and humans but rather with the reconciliation of the opposites within the God-image itself. Jung's approach here is psychological and not theological. His claim to be an agnostic (see chapter 5) is a statement about his relationship to theological statements or beliefs. When asked in a BBC interview whether he believed in God, Jung replied, "I do not believe, I know!"[14] By rooting his approach in the direct experience of knowing God rather than having a religion based on the affirmation of conceptual statements of belief, Jung was following an approach he first encountered in Eastern Yoga but later found to be also present in Western medieval alchemy.

In his commentary on *The Secret of the Golden Flower*, Jung summarized the significance of his encounter with Eastern religion as bringing God within the range of his own experience of reality. By this Jung did not mean that he was adopting the metaphysics or theology of Eastern religion, for this he explicitly rejects. However, by seeing God not as an absolute beyond all human experience, but as a powerful impulse within my personality, says Jung, "I must concern myself with him, for then he can become important even unpleasantly so, and can affect me in practical ways . . ."[15] Jung's theoretical explanation for this inner psychological experience of God rested upon his notion of the God archetype. This inherent God-image within each of us can have a unifying effect upon the whole personality. Especially noticeable is the way in which the opposing tensions are brought together by the guiding influence of the God archetype over the individual ego. In Jung's view, mysticism plays a large role in this whole process of uniting and balancing the opposing forces within experience. In this context, the term *mysticism* is being used, as just defined by Copleston, to mean the process of identifying with something more than the finite ego.

Mystical experiences, Jung felt, may have a powerful effect upon a person. The forces involved arise from the unconscious and transcend the finite ego so that, "He cannot grasp, comprehend, dominate them; nor can he free himself or escape from them, and therefore feels them as overpowering. Recognizing that they do not spring from his conscious personality, he calls them mana, daimon, or God."[16] Although these forces are nothing other than aspects of the unconscious, to call them merely "the unconscious," while empirically correct, would not be satisfactory for most people.

The mythic terms *mana*, *daimon*, or *God*, even though simply synonyms for the unconscious, prove to be especially effective in the production of mystical experience. The personification of the unconscious in such concepts enables an involvement of a wide range of emotions, for example, hate and love, fear and reverence. In this way, says Jung, the whole person is challenged and engaged.

> Only then can he become whole and only then can "God be born," that is, enter into human reality and associate with man in the form of "man." By this act of incarnation, man—that is, his ego—is inwardly replaced by "God," and God becomes outwardly man, in keeping with the saying of Jesus: 'Who sees me, sees the Father."[17]

For Jung the basic psychic process involved in the mystical experience is clearly the replacing of the conscious ego with the more powerful numinous forces of the unconscious that are called by the Western Christian "God." As to the content of these overpowering forces of the unconscious—the content of this 'God' concept—Jung is more explicit. The monotheism of Western religion and the all-encompassing absolute implied must be taken seriously. Within the one God must be found room for all the opposites encountered in experience, including even the opposites of good and evil. Only then, says Jung, will the unavoidable internal contradictions in the image of the creator-God be reconciled in the unity and wholeness of the self. "In the experience of the self it is no longer the opposites 'God' and 'man' that are reconciled, as it was before, but rather the opposites within the God-image itself."[18] Good and evil stand encompassed, held in tension, and transcended within the one absolute.

What is of interest for this discussion of mysticism is not so much the theological argument assumed, which Jung worked out in detail in his *Answer to Job*, but rather the psychological dynamics indicated. Jung's analysis shows mystical experience to occur when the finite, conscious ego is inwardly replaced by God, with God being understood as a personification of the numinous qualities of the unconscious. And here Jung is not making a metaphysical claim that God either exists or does not exist. Jung is simply observing that the processes involved in our experience of God are those of the unconscious. To put it simply, if we assume that God exists, then the way he acts upon us in overpowering mystical experiences is through the psychological processes of the unconscious, particularly via the God archetype.

A good illustration of this process is offered by Jung in his essay *The Holy Men of India*.[19] There Jung describes mysticism as the shifting of the center of gravity from the ego to the self, from man, as Jung puts it, to God. This, observes Jung, is the goal of *The Exercitia Spiritualia* of Ignatius Loyola: to subordinate "self-possession," or possession by an ego, as much as possible to possession by Christ.[20] Just as Christ manifests the reconciliation of the opposites within God's nature, so also does the person who surrenders his life to Christ overcome the conflict of the opposites within and achieves unity in God. As Jung puts it,

> God is the union of the opposites, the uniting of the torn asunder, the conflict is redeemed in the Cross. So Przywara says: "God appears in the cross," that is he manifests himself as the crucified Christ. The man who wishes to reach this unity in God,

> to make God real in himself, can only attain this through the Imitatio Christi, that is he must take up his cross and accept the conflict of the world and stand in the center of the opposites.[21]

For the Christian, God appears empirically in the suffering of the world, in the pain produced by the conflict between the opposites. One who would identify with God, therefore, does not seek to escape from the suffering of the world's conflicts, but rather gives up one's ego and identifies with Christ. By attempting to unite mystically with Christ, says Jung, "I enter the body of Christ through his scars, and my ego is absorbed into the body of Christ. Then like St. Paul, I no longer live but Christ lives in me."[22] Jung takes special care to urge that the preceding statement not be understood to mean identity, that "I am Christ," but rather only that, as Paul said it in *Galatians* 2:20, that He lives in us. In terms of psychological dynamics, the finite ego has been subordinated to the self.

A detailed description of the arising of the self in Jungian theory is rather complex and difficult. It is Jung's view that each of us shares in three different levels of consciousness: the conscious level of the ego; the dreams, memories, and repressions which comprise the personal unconscious; and the predispositions to universal human reactions, the archetypes, which compose the collective unconscious.[23] It is of course the notion of the archetypes and the collective unconscious which is the trademark of Jung's thought, and it is the idea of a "master archetype," namely, the "self" or "God" archetype, that is fundamental for Jung's analysis of mysticism.

Of all the archetypes, it is the self or God archetype which has the power to encompass all aspects of life in a way that is integrated and mature. To be comprehensive, both conscious stimuli from the external environment and internal impulses from within the personal and collective unconscious must be included. If one remains fixated on the conscious ego, its limited internal and external awareness will result in only a small portion of the stimuli available from all three levels of consciousness being included. In most ordinary experience there is only experience of the conscious level of ego awareness. Being grounded in the collective experience of humankind and being present within the unconscious of each person, the archetypes are the psychological mechanisms which enable us to get out from the too-narrow encapsulation of our conscious egos.

The archetypes are constantly trying to "raise up" or "reveal" some of the basic wisdom of humankind. But this requires the action of the thinking, feeling, sensing, and intuiting functions of the psyche. First there is the encounter of some external stimuli, for example, the seeing of an ordinary wooden cross on a building in a Christian culture. Initially the cross has no mystical significance and functions only at the ego-conscious level as a secular sign to designate the building as a church. But over the years as one matures, the cross image gradually acquires more significance and is carried, by the process of intuition, deeply into the psyche until the level of the collective unconscious is reached. There the God archetype, which has all the while been struggling upward to reveal itself, resonates sympathetically with the cross image and its Christian content of the crucified Christ. With the help of the other psychic functions—thinking, sensing, and feeling—the God archetype is given further individuation, using both the person's own creativity and the materials presented by a particular cultural tradition until the mystical revelation occurs.

Jung observes that initial indications often appear in dreams,[24] when the symbol being created first reaches the level of the personal subconscious. One becomes vaguely aware, perhaps for the first time, that the cross image is something much more than merely a sign to indicate that a building is a church. Rather than the church building, the cross and the figure of Christ simply being seen as routine parts of everyday life to be manipulated by the ego for its own purposes, the cross is now sensed as being numinous—as having a power and meaning about it which causes the conscious ego to pale by comparison. As the cross symbol becomes more complete, and the God archetype achieves full individuation at the level of conscious awareness, there occurs what Jung describes as a shift in the center of gravity within the psyche from the ego to the self. This is the mystical moment of illumination when the ego becomes aware of the larger and deeper collective dimension of consciousness and reality. In religious terms it may be variously described as a sudden or a gradual awakening in a moment of synchronicity.[25] But the key is that whereas previously things were experienced in a narrow egocentric way, now it is a sense of profound identity with the universal self which dominates. One is simultaneously united on the various levels within the psyche and taken out beyond the finite limitations of the ego. Thus, the mystical character of Jung's self-realization experience.

Although the cross and the crucified Christ are expected symbols of mystical self-realization in Christian cultures, Jung found the *maṇḍala* to be the most universal. As an image, it is the *maṇḍala's* characteristic of having an individualized center, yet expanding outward with the potential to include everything, that makes it a suitable symbol for mystical experience. Jung puts it as follows:

> The mandala's basic motif is the premonition of a center of personality, a kind of central point within the psyche, to which everything is related, by which everything is arranged, and which is itself a source of energy. . . . This center is not felt or thought of as the ego, but if one may so express it, as the *self.* Although the center is represented by an innermost point, it is surrounded by a periphery containing everything that belongs to the self—the paired opposites that make up the total personality. This totality comprises consciousness first of all, then the personal unconscious, and finally an indefinitely large segment of the collective unconscious whose archetypes are common to all mankind.[26]

Two things about the *maṇḍala* symbol impressed Jung. First, it occurred as a symbol for meditation in almost all great religions, and, in addition, it appeared independently in the dreams of his modern patients. Second the *maṇḍala* symbol wonderfully conveyed the sense of development around the center that included all sides and left nothing out. For Jung the *maṇḍala* was a pictorial representation of the circumambulation process of development which he took to be basic to the personality.[27]

Even though Jung felt that there were very definite differences between the mystical experiences of Eastern and Western religions, the psychological processes involved seemed very similar. Whereas in the East the *maṇḍala* served as a symbol both to clarify the nature of the deity philosophically and to aid in the development of that divine nature within one's own personality, so also the presentation and evoking of the proper relationship between God and man in Christian religion was expressed in the symbol of Christ or the cross.[28] In both cases the senses of completeness, union, and unity were highlighted, and these were universally reported as characteristics of mystical experience. In his *Commentary on the Secret of the Golden Flower*, Jung supported this contention of the commonness of mystical experience. He analyzed a mystical experience reported by Edward Maitland, the biographer of Anna Kingsford, and found in it the same sense of symbolic unity contained in the ancient Taoist Chinese text.[29]

While both Eastern and Western mysticism bear witness to the sense of transcendent unity that such philosophers as Walter Stace have called "the core of mysticism,"[30] Jung is very careful to make clear the subtle psychological differences in the way that unity is experienced: "Between the Christian and the Buddhist mandala there is a subtle but enormous difference. The Christian during contemplation would never say, 'I am Christ' but will confess with Paul, 'Not I, but Christ liveth in me.' [The Buddhist] sutra, however, says: 'Thou wilt know that thou art the Buddha.'"[31] At bottom both statements express a fundamental sense of unity, but in Jung's view, the way the unity is experienced is altogether different. The Buddhist statement "Thou art the Buddha" or the Hindu Upanisadic teaching "I am Brahman" requires complete removal of the individual ego or *ahaṃkāra*. The Western statement "Christ liveth in me" implies not a destruction of the ego but rather an invasion or possession by God so that the individual ego continues to exist only now as servant of the Lord. In mysticism, as in the other areas of psychological functioning, Jung simply would not accept the claim of Yoga thought that there could be conscious experience without a finite ego as the experiencer. As Jung saw it, the transcendent unity of the self needs the individual ego in order to be known, and the finite ego needs to be superceded by the transcendent self if integration and enlightenment are to occur.[32] From Jung's perspective a complementary relationship between the ego and the self, between the individual and the divine, is the necessary foundation for mystical experience. The mystical sense of the unity of the observer with all things requires an ego-observer as a basic prerequisite for that experience.

MYSTICISM IN THE YOGA PSYCHOLOGY OF PATAÑJALI

Patañjali's Yoga psychology approaches mysticism as a case of intuition, or supersensuous perception (*pratibhā*), from which distorting subjective emotions have been purged.[33] It will be recalled that the Western philosopher Stace defines mysticism in just such a perceptual way so as to avoid Russell's criticism that mystical experience is merely subjective emotion and as such has no direct touch with reality. Patañjali's claim is exactly the opposite. According to his Yoga psychology, mystical experience is a case of the direct supersensuous perception of reality, with various levels of mystical impurity being caused by obscuring emotions not yet purged from the perception. It is worth noting at the outset that in Yoga theory a major cause of obscuring emotion is the individual ego (*ahaṁkāra*)—the very aspect of the psyche that Jung felt to be essential.

Yoga psychology, following the Sāṅkhya theory of Indian philosophy,[34] conceives of consciousness as composed of three aspects, or substantive qualities (*guṇas*): *sattva* (brightness, illumination, intelligence), *rajas* (emotion, movement), and *tamas* (dullness, inertia). Although each of these *guṇas* keeps its own separate identity, no individual *guṇa* ever exists independently. Rather, the three *guṇas* are always necessarily found together like three strands of a rope. However, the proportionate composition of consciousness assigned to each of the *guṇas* is constantly changing.[35] Only the predominant *guṇa* will be easily recognized in a particular thought or perception. The other two *guṇas* will be present but subordinate, and therefore their presence will have to be determined by inference. If a "psychological cross-section" were taken through an ordinary state of consciousness, there would be a dominance of *tamas* and *rajas*, especially in its evolved forms of ego, sense organs, and their everyday experiences. In our routine states of consciousness, there is a noticeable lack of *sattva*, or pure discriminative awareness. However, in mystical experience the proportionate composition of consciousness by the *guṇas* is reversed, with *sattva* becoming dominant. At its height a pure *sattva* experience would be like the direct transparent viewing of reality with no emotional (*rajas*) or bodily (*tamas*) distortion intervening. This is technically termed *nirvicāra samādhi* in Indian mysticism, and is defined as a supernormal perception that transcends the ordinary categories of time, space, causality, and has the capacity to directly "grasp" or "see" the real nature of things.[36] It is this mystical experience of pure *sattva* intuition that is given detailed psychological analysis in *sūtras* I: 41–51 of Patañjali's *Yoga Sūtras*.

Patañjali begins his analysis with a general description of the mystical state of mind, which in Sanskrit is technically termed *samādhi*. In *samādhi* the mind (*citta*) is so intensely focused upon the object of meditation that the ordinary sense of the observer being separated from the object of study is overcome. There is a sense of being one with the object. As Patañjali puts it, it is as if the mind has become a transparent crystal that clearly reflects or transforms itself into the shape of the object being studied.[37] Vyāsa clarifies the intended meaning as follows: "As the crystal becomes colored by the color of the object placed beside it, and then shines according to the form of the object, so the mind is colored by the color of the object presented to it and then appears in the form of the object."[38] The ability of the mind to function in a crystal-like fashion requires a *sattva* dominance within consciousness.

The object referred to in this description may be any finite aspect of reality. The purpose of the object is simply to give the beginner a point of focus for his concentration, consequently it helps the process if the object exhibits a natural attractiveness to the student. One of the main tasks of the spiritual teacher, or *guru*, is to guide the student in selecting an object of meditation to the one that will be the most helpful. Since in Eastern thought it is generally held that the divine or absolute, whether it be conceptualized as Brahman, Buddha, Tao, or in some other form, is inherent in all of reality, therefore any aspect of reality may be suitably selected as an object for meditation. It may be some part of nature such as a flowing stream, it may be an image of Brahman, such as Lord Śiva or Mother Kāli, it may be the example set by the master Yogi Īśvara, or, at the most esoteric level, it may be nothing other than the flow of consciousness itself—mind (*citta*) taking itself as the object of its own meditation.[39] As we saw in our part I discussion of language, a word, verse, or linguistic symbol such as OM, when engaged in *mantra* chanting also functions in the same way. The process is not unlike that proposed by Jung where some object, such as a cross, provides the starting point for the subsequent individuation of the archetype into a symbol. However, it is immediately apparent that while both Patañjali and Jung begin with an object as a point of focus, Jung never leaves the object; it simply becomes transformed in one's experience from a surface sign to a deeply meaningful and in some sense universal symbol which mediates and integrates reality. Patañjali's Yoga, however, expects that the finite object, which is a limited symbol and therefore only partially able to mediate or manifest reality, must in the end be transcended. Only then can reality be fully "seen." It is this final state of unlimited congruence with reality (objectless *samādhi*) that is held by Patañjali to be the highest mystical state. And it is just such an attainment which Jung refuses to accept as possible, because it would require that the knowing ego, as one of the finite objects within consciousness, be transcended. In Jung's view, this results in a state with no knower to experience it, and therefore it is simply psychologically impossible. With this objection in mind, let us now examine Patañjali's description of the four levels of increasingly pure object *samādhi* and the final state of objectless *samādhi*, or the direct unlimited oneness with reality.

Of the four states of object *samādhi*, the lowest or most impure is called *savitarka*. It is impure, says Patañjali in *Yoga Sūtra* I: 42, because the *sattva* "reflection" of the object is obscured by a mixing up within consciousness of the following ingredients: the word (*Śabda*) used in conventional speech to label that object, the conceptual meaning (*artha*) of that object, and the direct perception (*jñāna*) of the object itself. Vyāsa explains that this mixed-up experience of the object has a twofold cause. On the one hand, there is the distortion caused by the habitual way in which word labels have been used to classify objects in this and previous lives. This has the mixing-up effect (*vikalpa*) within consciousness of causing our experience to be dominated by the conventional word labels of our language and culture (for example, saying "child," with the connotation "just another child") rather than by the perception of the object that is uniquely occurring at that moment (for example, "a brown-eyed child of a quiet, reflective mood with unfathomable beauty, dignity, and potential"). The other causes of *vikalpa*, or confusion, are the cognitive inferences based upon the conceptual meaning which the perception of the object evokes in our mind (for example, "a child is a gift of God to be treasured and loved" or "a child is a constant source of emotional frustration and a continuous drain upon the bank account"). Such cognitive inferences are either accepted from the traditional systems of thought of one's culture or belief (for example, a Christian view or a materialistic view) or may be made up by one's own imaginative thinking.[40] For most of us then, even when we manage to block out external distractions and concentrate sufficiently so as to become "caught up into oneness" with the object of our meditation, the kind of *samādhi* achieved is one that is obscured by the habitual way in which we give the object in view a word label ("stereotype it") and give it a biased or slanted coloring in our thinking.

In the second half of Vyāsa's commentary on *Yoga Sūtra* I: 42, the second level of object *samādhi* is defined as one in which the habitual patterns of past word usage and the biased patterns of inferential thinking are purged from the mind. Only then is the *sattva* or crystalline aspect of consciousness freed from the *rajas* or emotional obscuration so that "the object makes its appearance in the mind in its own distinct nature (unmixed up with word and meaning)."[41] The technical term for this state is *nirvitarka samādhi* and may be translated as "distinct mystical perception." It is this purified state of perception, says Vyāsa, that becomes the seed or basis for new verbal or inferential knowledge, namely, the truths taught by the mystics (*yogins*)—the truths they have learned from this higher form (*nirvitarka*) of perception. Vacaspati Miśra, in his gloss, points out that the yogi or mystic himself has no need to verbalize such truths, since he has it as a primary experience; for example, when you are hearing the greatness of the music, there is no need to try to verbalize that greatness in words. But because of compassion for others, the mystic speaks these truths, realizing however that the very speaking of them will necessarily add *rajas* or emotional distortion due to the usage of words and imagination.[42]

Whereas the two lower levels of object *samādhi* are based upon the gross or outer form of the object, the two higher levels are directed toward the inner essence—what might today be called the atomic or microcosmic structure of the object. Descriptions of such states are offered in *Yoga Sūtras* I: 43 and 44, although the distinctions become so subtle as to virtually deify conceptualization. The third level is called *savicāra samādhi*. In *savicāra* experience, the flow of consciousness so completely identifies with the object alone that the mind is as it were "devoid of its own nature."[43] I take Vyāsa to mean by this that there is a complete loss of ego-consciousness. This does not mean one lapses into some sort of stupor. On the contrary, what is implied is that one is so "caught-up" in the object that there is no room left for a separate awareness of one's own ego as the thing that is having the experience. One has forgotten oneself. The object in all its vividness of both external characteristics and internal qualities totally commands one's attention. The only distinguishing characteristics given to the experience are provided by the object itself. In the *savicāra* state, awareness of the object includes both its gross form and its microcosm or inner essence but is limited in space and time to the present. The yogin's knowledge ("knowing by becoming one with") of the object is complete, but it is knowledge only as of the present moment in space and time.

Nirvicāra, or the final stage of object *samādhi*, differs only from *savicāra* in that in the *nirvicāra* the limitation to the present moment in space and time is overcome. Now the *yogin* is so completely one with the object that he is one with all its past states, as well as its present moment, and shares fully in the various possibilities of the future. The last limitations of space and time are transcended. According to Vyāsa, a mystical state reaches the *nirvicāra* level when it is, as it were, void of its own nature and becomes the object itself. This is the highest level of knowledge of a finite object which may be reached. An example of such a *nirvicāra* state might be the knowledge that a lover of a particular person realizes when the other person is so completely known that, as we put it, "they are like an open book." In the Christian tradition, one might identify the knowledge Amos had of Israel,[44] Jesus had of the Samaritan woman at the well,[45] or St. Francis had of the animals. Mystical experience of this sort is far from being misty, vague, or mysterious. It is as vivid and immediate as is possible for one who habitually lives at the lower levels of awareness to imagine. Its psychological nature would, as Stace suggested, seem to approximate that of sense perception—only on a supernormal level. From the perspective of Patañjali's Yoga psychology, the two highest levels of object *samādhi* are characterized by a complete self-forgetting or egolessness. The mystic consciousness has so fully become one with the object that it no longer appears as an object of consciousness. The duality of subject and object is overcome, leaving only the steady transformation of pure *sattva* consciousness into the form of the object, allowing the thing-itself (*svarūpa*) to shine forth in itself alone.[46]

The highest level of mystical realization in Patañjali's yoga is reached when even the limitation of focusing on a finite object is left behind. *Yoga Sūtras* I: 50 and 51 describe the establishment of "seedless," or objectless, *samādhi*. No longer does the yogin meditate on an object, not even such an exhalted object as the Lord himself. Now consciousness turns in upon itself and becomes one with its own self-luminous nature. According to both Sāṅkhya theory and Yoga psychology, in this state there is only pure knowing consciousness. The lower "filtering organs" of ego (*ahaṁkāra*), mind, and sense organs with their component *rajas* or emotion have been dropped off or transcended. There remains only the pristine existence of reality itself, which is revealed to be nothing other than the pure discriminative consciousness of the true self (*puruṣa*).[47]

In agreement with the authors previously discussed, Patañjali, although very familiar with psychic powers (*siddhis*) such as levitation,[48] warns against confusing such attainments with true mystical experiences. Special powers may be produced by drugs, by fasting, or as side effects of true spiritual meditation. Consequently, the *yogin* or mystic must be constantly on guard against the temptation to use such powers, as will naturally come to one, for one's own fame and fortune. To do that, says Patañjali, would only further attachment to egoic states such as pride, greed, and fear—opposites of a true mystical experience.

THE PSYCHOLOGIES OF JUNG AND PATAÑJALI COMPARED

The preceding review of Jungian psychology and Patañjali's Yoga shows both points of agreement and difference. Both authors agree with the definition of mystical experience presented by the philosophers at the outset as being characterized by a loss of the sense of finite ego and a corresponding increased identification with a transcendent spiritual reality. But there was definite disagreement about the degree of ego loss which occurs and about the kind of psychological process which is mainly responsible for the mystic's identification with the larger transcendent reality.

With regard to the degree of ego loss involved, it was Jung's view that in mystical experience there was a replacing of the conscious ego with the more powerful numinous forces of the unconscious arising from the God or self archetype. As he put it, there is a shifting of the center of gravity within the personality from ego to self, from man to God. This shift of the center resulted in more of the sum total of reality being experienced and included within the personality. The mystical experience is comprehensive of both conscious stimuli from the external environment and internal impulses from within the personal and collective unconscious. This breadth of awareness means that one participates in the conflicts of the opposing forces which constitute the world. In the Christian context, this is expressed as the suffering of Christ and is symbolized by the cross. The ego loss envisaged by Jung is the loss required so that one could say with Paul, "It is no longer I who live, but Christ who lives in me." The ego has not been totally lost or discarded but merely made into a servant of the Lord.

Jung correctly recognized that there was a fundamental disagreement between himself and Patañjali over the degree of ego loss involved in mystical experience. Whereas in Jung's view the mystical experience of reality required the continued existence of an ego in order to be known, for Patañjali's Yoga the ego was nothing more than a limiting and distorting emotional obscuration which had to be removed if the real was to be fully known. In the two lower states of *savitarka-* and *nirvitarka-samādhi*, the presence of ego and its habitually limiting ways of perceiving and thinking rendered the mystical experience impure. However, in the higher states of *savicāra-* and *nirvicāra-samādhi*, the mind by virtue of being completely devoid of its own ego is able to be perfectly transparent to the object being meditated upon. Such complete and direct experience of some objective aspect of reality requires that the mystic not allow his or her own ego and mental processes to get in the way. Although Patañjali, with his requirement for a complete negation of ego, has already gone well beyond Jung's more limited Western point of view, the ultimate state has still to be reached according to Yoga. In addition to the limiting factor of the individual ego being removed, the full mystic experience requires that reality be experienced in its completeness and not in just the limited form of a finite object as one point of meditation. For the Yoga point of view, even if the object of one's meditation be an incarnation of the divine, the Lord himself, something of the fullness of reality will have been "dropped off" to enable the limited incarnation to take place. Thus, for Patañjali, it is the objectless *samādhi*, in which consciousness becomes one with its own self-luminous nature, that is the highest mystical experience. It is such an experience that is indicated by phrases such as "I am Brahman" or "I am Buddha," and that differs so radically from the Christian "Christ lives in me."

With regard to the kind of psychological processes involved, Jung seems to follow the lead of Rudolf Otto and William James, whereas Patañjali is much closer to the approach suggested by Walter Stace. In Jung's analysis, mystical experience, although it may begin with intuition, necessarily also involves the other psychological processes of feeling, thinking, and sensing. For Patañjali, the processes of emotion and thinking had to be purged until only pure perception remained. Jung, to a large extent, followed Otto's suggestion of an analogy to aesthetic experience. Patañjali, like Stace, appealed to the model of sense perception. Jung followed James in pointing to the unconscious as the locus of mystical experience; for Yoga the opposite condition of complete consciousness is identified as the mystical.

In the face of the earlier comparative psychological study, we find ourselves left with what is perhaps a new and expanded version of Stace's question, "Does mystical experience point to an objective reality or is it merely a subjective phenomenon?" Now the psychological question must be added, "Can there be mystical experience without an individual ego?" Or put another way, "Is unlimited consciousness of the fullness of reality psychologically possible?" This question will be given further discussion in the following chapter on Yoga and the transpersonal psychologists.

8

The Limits of Human Nature in Yoga and Transpersonal Psychology

Views of the limits and perfectibility of human nature differ fundamentally between much of Eastern and Western thought. This fact is especially evident when the Yoga psychologies of the East are compared with the transpersonal psychologies of the West. Transpersonal psychologists, such as Carl Jung, are greatly drawn to Yoga psychology and influenced by it, as we have shown in chapters 6 and 7. Yet even they draw a clear line beyond which they will not go, namely, the Yoga claim that human nature is not finite, that its ego limitations can be transcended to the point of perfection. In Jung's view, as we saw in the previous chapter, it is simply not psychologically possible to dispense with the knowing ego, as Yoga claims to do. Total overcoming of the ego would result not in omniscience—the Yoga claim—but in a state of unconsciousness, since there would not be an ego to experience anything. In drawing this firm line against the Yoga claims of the perfectibility or limitlessness of human nature, Jung is paralleling Kant's claim that, in terms of epistemology, human nature is finite—it can never know "the thing itself"—and the theological claim of Christianity that human nature is fatally flawed.[1]

While these conflicting assessments of the perfectibility of human nature await a definitive study, a number of recent books have begun to lay the groundwork for a solution. The opportunity for Western scholars to understand the Yoga claims is advanced by the availability in English translation of Jean Varenne's *Yoga and the Hindu Tradition*.[2] While the translation of Patañjali's *Yoga Sūtras* has been available in English for many years, it is set in the esoteric conventions of aphorisms and commentaries that characterized the scholarly style of early classical India. Consequently it is difficult for the modern mind to appropriate. Eliade opened it to the West in his 1954 *Le Yoga: Immortalité et Liberté* (translated by Willard Trask and published in 1958 as *Yoga: Immortality and Freedom*). While he gives much helpful clarification of esoteric terms and practices, Eliade concludes his study by observing that, when it comes to the Yoga ideal of a perfected state (the *jīvan-mukta*) in which no personal consciousness exists but only omniscient awareness, "We shall not attempt to describe this paradoxical condition; indeed, since it is obtained by 'death' to the human condition and rebirth to a transcendent mode of being, it cannot be reduced to our categories."[3]

Like Eliade, Varenne finds the texts describing the perfected Yogi to be paradoxical. Although the individual ego-personality is claimed to have been transcended, the Yogi does not vanish, as the *Yoga Sūtras* and other such texts logically suggest should happen. To continue with a physical body and all its sensory and cognitive limitations does not square with the claims of omniscience, and omnipresence that we find in the *Yoga Sūtras*. The usual response to this paradox in the Yoga texts is that while there is no necessity for the perfected yogi to retain a body, he or she does so only for the purpose of helping others, such as students, reach that same perfected state—the goal of all religion, philosophy, and psychology.

As *jīvan-mukti*, or "living liberation," is a unique idea in Hindu thought, let us take a moment to examine it in more detail. The *jīvan-mukti* tradition has a long and highly respected parentage. From Śaṅkara (c. 700 CE) to contemporary scholars (e.g., Sarvepali Radhakrishnan) and saints (e.g., Ramana Maharshi or Sri Aurobindo) varying interpretations of the idea are found. In his authoritative studies, Andrew Fort finds that while most agree that salvation or release can be realized in this life, there is no consensus on exactly what one is liberated from or to.[4] Fort notes, "In addition to disputes about the possibility of embodied liberation, there are differing views on the types, degrees, or stages of liberation, some attainable in the body and some not."[5] One thing is common, however, namely that all experiences of ego-sense must be transcended for the realization of the *jīvan-mukti* state. This is where the *jīvan-mukti* idea connects with the discussion of this chapter over the very possibility of an egoless state. Western thought rejects the idea of egolessness, whereas the Yoga psychology of Patañjali assumes its necessity for release from rebirth (*saṁsāra*). The *jīvan-mukti* notion goes further in providing detailed description and discussion of exactly what such an egoless state of salvation or release is like when experienced before death. In fact a classical Hindu text of the fourteenth century CE, the *Jīvan-Mukti-Viveka* of Vidyāraṇya, offers a systematic analysis of the evidence for the state of living liberation while in the body, its psychological make-up, and its purpose.[6] The text specifically distinguishes between the more usual Western notion of liberation after death through release from the body and the *jīvan-mukti* state of liberation while still alive and embodied. Patricia Mumme[7] notes that the seed ideas of the *jīvan-mukti* notion are found in several passages of the *Upaniṣads*, the basic texts of Hindu scripture. She suggests the Buddhists may have contributed the idea that release from *karma* could be achieved in a living state called *nirvāṇa*, and this helped to inspire development of a parallel concept in Hindu thought. A foundational text of the Sāṅkhya School, the *Sāṃkhya Kārikā*, proposed the analogy of the potter's wheel to help explain how embodiment could continue in a *karma*-free, egoless, liberated, and enlightened person. The analogy runs as follows. Just as when the potter finishes making a pot, the wheel continues from its own inertia to turn a few more revolutions, so also the body of one who has realized release, that is, has removed all *karma* and ego-sense, continues on for a while—a few more revolutions as it were—out of its own inertia, offering the opportunity to be a *guru* and teach others. Among the Hindu schools, the Advaita

Vedānta has made the most use of the *jīvan-mukti* concept and has continued its development right up to the present.[8] Indeed the contemporary neo-Vedantists, in seeking to engage current ideas of ecumenism and social concern for all with traditional *jīvan-mukti* thinking, have made the concept into a universal truth that holds for all, thus directly challenging more limited Western views of the perfectibility of human nature. The neo-Vedantists even offer the contemporary example of the Hindu saint, Ramana Maharshi, as a twentieth century *jīvan-mukta*, or one who has achieved liberation while embodied.[9]

Returning to the *Yoga Sūtras*, it is clear there that through practice of the eight steps (*Yogāṅga*) the karmic obscurations or *saṁskāras* (memory traces) that obstruct liberation or release from rebirth can be gradually diminished. Through intense Yogic meditation (*tapas*) these seed states (*bigās*), as the text calls them, can be "burned up" and removed from the flow of consciousness.[10] When the last *saṁskāra* is burnt up, then one is released from rebirth and omniscience is realized. The potter's wheel analogy is employed to explain why, once release is realized, one retains a body at all. The example offered in the text of one who exemplifies this state is Īśvara, the master yogi who all devotees are to emulate. And, as Chapple notes, the modern Yoga commentator Hariharananda Aranya calls this the state of *jīvanmukti*.[11]

Even before reaching the ultimate point, the *Yoga Sūtras* provide a detailed technical description of four levels of direct knowing that transcend subject-object separation.[12] These four levels of object *samādhi* were given detailed discussion in the previous chapter. While much of our daily experience is characterized by experiences in which we, as the subjects, examine objects that are separate from us, we all have experiences in which we seem to lose our sense of separation and are caught up into the object, as when we "lose ourselves" in sexual orgasm, in the hearing of music, in the seeing of a sunset, or in the moment of religious devotion. The *Yoga Sūtra* analysis of such union or object-*samādhi* experiences is theoretically sophisticated and cannot be easily dismissed. Yet it clearly transcends our normal Western understanding of the limits of perception and cognition that characterize human nature. For the contemporary reader, Varenne provides a fully contextualized presentation of Yoga that is interesting and readable.

While most Yoga claims regarding subject-object or ego transcendence are scorned by mainstream North American psychology, a small group of thinkers study the Eastern texts and go some distance toward accepting the Yoga claims. They are the transpersonal psychologists, so called because they argue that humans are capable of transcending their personal limitations to varying degrees. Andrew Fort suggests that the transpersonal psychologists are showing some understanding and acceptance of Eastern thought.

> One piece of evidence is the frank acknowledgment that therapy (developing the ego-self) is not the same as liberation (insight into the falsity of the ego-self). Having a "well-adjusted" ego structure is different from transcending one's identity; to *Advaitins*, "identity" in this sense is an obstacle, the source of ignorance of true identity with unlimited pure consciousness. As "to be nice is not to be saved," so to be "together" is not to be liberated.[13]

Just how far do the transpersonal psychologists extend the limits of human nature? Michael Washburn, in *The Ego and the Dynamic Ground,* sets forth a new paradigm for psychological development that bridges Freud and Jung and draws on both Eastern and Western religions.[14] Washburn's thesis is that "the ego, as ordinarily constituted, can be transcended and that a higher, trans-egoic plane or stage of life is possible."[15] This higher stage is reached when the ego is properly rooted in its Dynamic Ground, which for Washburn is the psychological locus of the divine. Washburn presents his theory over against the transpersonal theory of Ken Wilbur and in contrast to the structural-hierarchial paradigms of Piaget and Kohlberg. Washburn's theory is dynamic, triphasic, and dialectic: dynamic, in that the primary focus is on the ego's interaction with the Dynamic Ground; triphasic, in that human development is seen as occurring in three principal stages: (1) pre-egoic, a period in which the Dynamic Ground dominates a weak and underdeveloped ego, (2) egoic, latter childhood and middle adulthood, when the ego dissociates itself from the Dynamic Ground through repression to make growth possible, and (3) trans-egoic or latter adulthood, in which a strong and matured ego is integrated with the Dynamic Ground; and *dialectical,* in that progress through the stages is not straightforward but a back-and-forth process of negation of the Ground, return to the Ground, and a final trans-egoic integration.

Washburn has simplified Freud's id, ego, and superego by removing the superego and reinterpreting the id by adding to it positive elements of the divine, like Jung's God archetype or the Hindu self *(ātman,* the divine within one). What results is a bipolar psyche consisting of ego and Dynamic Ground that interact in different ways at each stage of development. Washburn sides with Freud against Jung in his retention of repression and regression as the major psychological mechanisms for maturation. Unlike Freud, however, here "regression is in service of transcendence."[16] For Washburn, personality development begins in a period of dialectical conflict between the dominant Dynamic Ground (symbolized as the Great Mother and the Oedipal Father) and the weak ego, which is attempting to strengthen and grow. This the ego does by dissociating itself, through repression, from its Dynamic Ground so as to create a mental ego. Although freed from domination by the Dynamic Ground, the mental ego experiences the existential anguish of alienation, guilt, and despair. Unlike the existentialists who take such anguish to be the essence of the human condition, Washburn sees it as a necessary but passing phase that sets the stage for the growth of self through the regression of the mental ego to its true foundation in the Dynamic Ground. At this point, Washburn is strongly influenced by Jung's notion of the individuation of the God, or self, archetype as being the height of personality development. He suggests that meditation is an aid to this process and identifies two types: concentrative, such as Patañjali's Yoga, and reflective, such as Jung's active imagination, and suggests that prayer can be of either type.

When it comes to the crucial question of the degree to which transcendence of the ego is possible, Washburn remains resolutely Western and rooted in a Jewish or Christian position. Through "regression in the service of transcendence," the mental ego gives up its autonomy and opens itself by regression to recover its roots in the Dynamic

Ground. This leads to integration of the instincts, the body, and the external world in experiences of awe, ecstasy, blessedness, and bliss. A weakness of this otherwise original and creative approach is that discussion of the final achievements of integration, such as prophetic vision, saintly compassion, and mystical illumination, are given only minimal development. Washburn adopts a negative assessment of the possibility of egoless and objectless states of concentration (the Yoga claim). It is clear that for him human nature is limited; transcendence reaches its height in the degree to which the ego by surrendering its autonomy is infused and illumined by the divine spirit of the Dynamic Ground. But the ego itself can never be completely transcended.

Alan Roland sees the transcendence of the individual embodied in Yoga psychology from the quite different perspective of the "extended self." In his *In Search of Self in India and Japan*, Roland demonstrates that the concept of 'self' varies radically according to culture.[17] In the modern West it is the highly individualized self that enables one to function in a society that emphasizes personal autonomy. The modern Western self is characterized by "I-ness," has self-contained outer boundaries, sharply differentiates between self and others, and has narcissistic structures of self-regard. The ideal is seen in terms of varying degrees of individualism from competitiveness to self-actualization. When Roland, a New York psychiatrist, attempted to apply therapeutic theories based upon these Western concepts (e.g., Freud, Erikson, Hartman) to patients from India, he found that they did not work because a different conception of human nature and self was operative.

Indian patients in both New York and India manifested an extended view of human nature and a familial sense of self. Within the extended family, there is constant interchange through permeable ego boundaries and high levels of empathy and receptivity to others. The experiential sense of self is the "We-Self" rather than the "I-Self." The ideal is focused not on the individual self but on the self of the hierarchical extended family and ultimately on the universal spiritual self (*ātman*) that is within everyone. For this spiritualized self to be realized, particular mental structures of the individual must be dismantled until only pure consciousness remains.[18] This, says Roland, is the exact opposite of the West, where the aim is the pursuit and proliferation of mental structures as unifiers of reality. For the Indian mind, there is no ultimate subject-object duality; nature is to be lived in, not mastered. The end goal is the transforming of the subjective consciousness rather than the exercise of our specific mental structures in controlling the environment. By contrast, the Western mind takes a fundamental dualism between subject and object to be universally valid. Knowledge is pursued to discover the conceptual unity behind the diverse phenomena. The overall goal is to control the object rather than to change the subject—the goal of Indian Yoga disciplines. It is clear that according to Roland, views of human nature are strongly culturally conditioned, and the individualistic limits that typify Western experience cannot be assumed to be universal. Roland shows that psychological structuring is embedded in distinct views of human nature, social patterns, and childrearing practices of various cultures.

Roland's book adds crucial psycho-social dimensions to our study of Yoga, religion, and our general view of human nature. It catches vital nuances of self-experience that escape philosophical and historical approaches. Roland's analysis of Indian spiritual experience is somewhat simplistic, is overly influenced by Vedānta philosophy, and shows no sensitivity to the cultural diversity within India. Yet in spite of these limitations, Roland's book opens important new ground; Roland lead us to question further any assumptions regarding the limited or unlimited character of human nature. As he effectively demonstrates, all such assumptions are culturally conditioned.

In the 1970s, a series of books established a new movement in the field of psychology called "transpersonal psychology." This movement was concerned with integrating Yoga and modern Western psychology, as well as with exploring the limits of human nature. During the decade of the 1970s, Charles Tart was the leading figure in this group of thinkers, and his book, *Transpersonal Psychologies*, is their key statement.[19] In many ways they were more open to Yoga and its challenge to Western views of human limitations than thinkers such as Jung and Washburn were. It will be of interest to see how far the transpersonalists were willing to push the limits of the West in opening up to the claims of Yoga psychology.

Tart begins by positioning transpersonal psychology within modern psychological thought as follows: "Transpersonal Psychology," says Tart, "is the title given to an emerging force in the psychology field by a group of psychologists . . . who are interested in those *ultimate* human capacities and potentialities that have no systematic place in behaviouristic theory . . . , classical psychoanalytic theory . . . , or humanistic psychology."[20] States such as mystical or unitive experiences, awe, bliss, and transcendence of the self are pointed to as the contents to be studied by transpersonal psychology. A leading transpersonal psychologist, Robert Ornstein, in his *The Nature of Human Consciousness*, argues for the asking of such fundamental questions as "Is consciousness individual or cosmic?" and "What means are there to extend human consciousness?"[21] To answer these questions, Ornstein suggests, modern Western psychology needs to link up with the esoteric psychologies of other cultures, such as the Yoga psychology of Patañjali). Tart attempts a beginning to such answers in his *Transpersonal Psychologies* by treating modern Western psychology as just one among many psychologies. So after outlining the assumptions of modern Western empirical psychology in chapter 2, he goes on to include what he calls the traditional or esoteric "spiritual psychologies," including Buddhist, Sufi, Christian, and Hindu Yoga, in succeeding chapters.

In the Yoga chapter, written by Haridas Chaudhuri, the development of the personality from infancy is described as punctuated by changing patterns of self-image or self-identity.

> When the growing infant becomes aware of himself as an individual entity separate from the mother, he identifies himself with the body. This is his material self (*annamaya purusha*). Next, he identifies himself with his vital nature—that is with various impulses, passions, and desires. This is his vital self (*pranamaya purusha*). Next he identifies himself with his mental nature as a sentient percipient being (*manomaya purusha*). This is his aesthetic nature. Next he identifies himself with his rational nature and perceives himself as a thinking, deliberating, choosing being (*vijnanamaya purusha*). Finally, through a bold meditative breakthrough in conscious-

> ness he discovers the transcendental level of existence and finds his true self there (*anandamaya purusha*).[22]

It is this final "bold breakthrough" that is questioned by Western psychologists as stretching the limits of human nature beyond the possible. Yet it is just that breakthrough of ego-limitations to transcendent consciousness that is taken to be the goal of life by Yoga and the other Eastern psychologies and religions. Yoga describes this "transcendent consciousness" as a deeper level beyond the subject-object dichotomy and beyond the limitations of a filtering individual ego—a level of pure transcendence experienced as the great Silence, as the unutterable Peace that passeth understanding. "The dichotomy of subject and object, spectator and spectacle, witness and his field of observation, is entirely dissolved. The silent Self shines as the absolute (*kevala*)."[23] Here Chaudhuri is describing the *nirvikalpa samādhi* state of Patañjali's Yoga outlined in the previous chapter. It is the question as to whether such a state of altered consciousness is in reality the goal to be achieved by all of us, through repeated rebirths, until it is realized (the Yoga claim) or whether Eastern intuition has overreached itself and is suggesting a goal that may be imagined but is not realizable (as Jung, Washburn, Passmore, and other Western thinkers have claimed).

John Hick, the scholar of comparative philosophy and religion, has taken up the question afresh. In his recent book, *The Fifth Dimension*, Hick shows himself most open to the claims of the mystics of all traditions. However, in response to the Yoga and other claims of "union with the Ultimate in this life" Hick argues that such claims must be understood "metaphorically" rather than "literally." Like Jung, Hick argues that if indeed "the finite consciousness of the mystic had been dissolved in the Infinite, like a drop of water becoming part of the ocean, there would be no unbroken thread of finite consciousness continuing through the experience and subsequently able to recall it. Thus it seems to me that if individual identity is indeed lost in the ocean of Brahman, this must be a state from which there is no return, and hence no possibility of its being reported by a still living mystic."[24] Consequently, in Hick's view, any such mystical reports must not be taken as "literal" but as "metaphorical" in nature.

In my view, the open-minded approach of Tart, Ornstein, and the transpersonal psychologists of the 1970s has more to offer than Hick's interpretation. Rather than taking as absolute truth the Western presuppositions that our human nature is limited by its finite, individual ego and therefore incapable of realizing the various levels of *samādhi* that Patañjali's Yoga describes, we should adopt a critical, curious, and openminded approach to Yoga and its claims. Indeed, Vachaspati Mishra's *Gloss* on *Yoga Sūtra* IV: 25 offers an explanation of such doubters of Yoga: "For one who does not ponder at all upon the existence of the self, the heretic [who has not practiced the eight aids to yoga under a guru in this or a previous life]—for him . . . not seeing the distinction, there is no cessation of pondering upon the existence of the self."[25] Stuck in endless questioning and failing to practice Patañjali's eight steps of Yoga, the doubter naturally does not see the cessation of mental fluctuation claimed by Yoga to be a real possibility. Thus, the Yoga tradition itself anticipates Hick's "metaphorical rather than literal" move and explains it as the expected psychological state of one who has not seriously taken up the practice of Yoga under a qualified teacher. Such a person, claims Yoga, is in no position to pass judgment on whether or not such states, such as egolessness, are psychologically possible. The transpersonal psychologists remain open to the possibility that such states may be realizeable and thus show scholarly respect for the Yoga tradition of India. The dominant Western view of the psychological, epistemological, and spiritual limits of human nature needs careful, critical re-examination, as do the Yoga claims of the human capacity for complete psychological and spiritual union with the divine.

9

conclusion

The *Yoga Sūtras* of Patañjali, India's traditional psychology, have been shown to be foundational for the Indian understanding of how language functions both in ordinary communication and in the *mantra* chanting to achieve release (*mokṣa*). Yoga psychology has also been seen to influence modern psychologists, including Carl Jung and the transpersonalists such as Charles Tart. However, both Jung and the transpersonalists were found to have a fundamental disagreement with the ultimate claims of Yoga psychology that has important implications for our understanding of the limits of human nature.

The philosophy of language and theology of revelation of the great Indian grammarian Bhartṛhari was shown in part I to be made more understandable and practicable when undergirded by Patañjali's Yoga psychology. From the everyday experience of ordinary language to the experience of scripture as divine revelation, the philosophy and poetry of Bhartṛhari is made more credible when interpreted through the psychological processes of Patañjali's Yoga. This book's contribution is its demonstration that Bhartṛhari knew Patañjali's Yoga psychology and assumed it in his own thinking. For the modern reader, knowing something of Patañjali's Yoga helps us to understand the Eastern claim that language, especially the language of scriptures such as the Vedas or syllables like AUM/OM, when chanted as *mantras* have power to remove obstructions (*karma*) from consciousness until release or union with the divine is realized.

Turning to modern Western psychology, we observed parallels between the thinking of Freud and Jung on memory and the Yoga conception of *karma*. We saw that the traditional Yoga explanation of memory in terms of how the *guṇas*, or constituents of consciousness, function in various karmic states closely parallels contemporary ideas, such as Eccles's experiments on memory and motivation. The Yoga psychology notion of *vāsanās*, or habit patterns, as resulting from repetitions of a particular memory trace, or *saṁskāra*, fits well with the modern idea of growth at the synaptic spines. We saw that both Yoga and Freud agreed that memory and motivation are parts of a single psychic process which also embodies choice, but disagreed as to the degree to which this choice process is free or determined. Yoga psychology goes much further than Freud in providing for free choice and for the possibility that the processes of memory and motivation can be transcended.

Unlike Freud, Carl Jung learned some Sanskrit, read the *Yoga Sūtras* for himself, and gave lectures on them. We demonstrated how Jung's thinking on memory, perception, and knowledge was influenced and supported by Yoga, but more importantly, where he drew the line in his acceptance of Patañjali's psychology. As we saw in chapter 6, Jung argued that Patañjali's failure to distinguish between philosophy and psychology led to Yoga's over-reaching of itself, as Jung put it, as, for example, in the Yoga claim that the individual ego can be completely transcended and union with pure consciousness realized, as in the Buddha's enlightenment experience. Jung felt that this Yoga claim was a psychological projection of an idea that could not be embodied in human experience. Yet something like this conception of union with the divine is exactly what is claimed by the mystics, especially in the East. Using the psychologies of both Jung and Yoga, we showed how such mystical experience can be given detailed explanation in terms of psychological process, but with very different assessments as to the nature and degree of ego-transcendence claimed and achieved.

The ongoing argument between traditional Yoga and modern Western psychology over the limits of human nature was further explored in our discussion of the transpersonal psychologists and the comparative philosopher John Hick. While Yoga psychology and Eastern thought in general clearly claim that the autonomous individual can and must be transcended for the fullness of life to be achieved, the Western view is that human nature is finite, limited, and not capable of being opened up by Yoga practices of language, such as *mantra* chanting, or meditation until union with the divine is realized. In Jung's view any practice leading to transcendence of the individual ego, to the extent that it is possible, will result in the person falling into an unconscious state—not enlightenment. The Western philosopher John Hick discounts such Yoga claims as being simply metaphors and not be taken as claims to literal truth. Yet there is no question that the psychological processes described in the *Yoga Sūtras* are meant to be taken literally, not metaphorically, as the development of the *jīvanmukti* (living liberation) tradition in India demonstrates. The transpersonal psychologists examined showed varying degrees of openness to the radical nature of this Yoga claim.

I do not come down on one side or the other in this fundamentally important debate over the limits of human nature—but I find myself fascinated by it. My contention is that good comparative scholarship requires that we examine such claims within the presuppositions of their own worldviews. There is no theological, philosophical, or psychological helicopter that will get us above all biases or assumptions so as to decide which are right or wrong. Therefore, as scholars, we must remain critical but open. And to critically test the claims of Yoga, say the *Yoga Sūtras*, one must first try to master it under the guidance of a teacher or *guru*. Only then would one be in a position to conclude, as Jung and Hick do, that the states of consciousness described in the *Yoga Sūtras* are, when taken literally, beyond the possibilities of human experience. Our study of Patañjali's *Yoga Sūtras* has clearly focused the parameters of this debate—in language and psychology—that is at the root of the disagreement as to the limits of human nature between Eastern and Western thought. This debate has profound implications for psychology, philosophy, and theology and is deserving of further study. It is the subject of my next book.

notes

CHAPTER ONE
INTRODUCTION

1. J. H. Woods, *The Yoga-System of Patañjali*. Delhi: Motilal Banarsidass, 1966, p. xix for the date offered by Woods.

2. David M. Rosenthal (ed.), *The Nature of Mind*. New York: Oxford University Press, 1991.

3. Ned Block, Owen Flanagan, and Gwen Guzeldere (eds.), *The Nature of Consciousness*. Cambridge, Mass.: M.I.T. Press, 1997.

4. Jadunath Sinha, *Indian Psychology: Cognition*. Calcutta: Sinha Publishing House, 1958, pp. 334–366.

5. See Mircea Eliade, *Yoga: Immortality and Freedom*. Trans. by Willard R. Trask. Princeton: Princeton University Press, 1971, p. 5, and T. H. Stcherbatsky, *The Conception of Buddhist Nirvāṇa*. London: Mouton, 1965, pp. 16–19.

6. *Patañjaliyogadarsanam*. Varanasi: Bharatīya Vidyā Prakāśana, 1963. For a readable English translation, see Rama Prasada, *Patañjali's Yoga Sūtras*. Allahabad: Bhuvaneswari Asrama, 1924. More recent translations include Bengali Baba, *The Yogasūtra of Patañjali*. Delhi: Motilal Banarsidass, 1976, and Georg Feuerstein, *The Yoga-Sūtra of Patañjali*. Folkestone, Kent: Dawson, 1979. A good recent secondary source on the Yoga school is Ian Whicher, *The Integrity of the Yoga Darśana*. Albany: State University of New York Press, 1998. Gerald Larson is editing the "Yoga" volume of the *Encyclopedia of Indian Philosophies* published by Motilal Banarsidass, but it is not yet available. For the Sāṅkhya background assumed by the Yoga school, see G. Larson and R. S. Bhattacharya (eds.), *Sāṁkhya: A Dualist Tradition in Indian Philosophy*, Vol. IV, Encyclopedia of Indian Philosophies. Delhi: Motilal Banarsidass, 1987.

7. For a detailed study of this approach, see Harvey Alper (ed.), *Understanding Mantras*. Albany: State University of New York Press, 1989.

8. See, for example, Bruce K. Alexander, "The Roots of Addiction in Free Market Society," *Canadian Centre for Policy Alternatives*, April 2001, Vancouver, B.C.: www.policyalternatives.ca.bc/rootsofaddiction.html.

9. Rudolf Otto, *The Idea of the Holy*. Oxford: Oxford University Press, 1977.

10. John Hick, *The Fifth Dimension*. Oxford: Oneworld, 1999, pp. 136 ff.

11. See, for example, John Passmore, *The Perfectibility of Man*. New York: Charles Scribner's Sons, 1970.

CHAPTER TWO
ĀGAMA IN THE
YOGA SŪTRAS OF PATAÑJALI

1. Pamela McCallum, "Editorial," Issues of Language volume of *Ariel, 15*, 1984, p. 8.

2. *Yogadarśanam of Patañjali*. Varanasi: Bharatīya Vidyā Prakāsana, 1963. English translations referred to include *The Yoga System of Patañjali*, trans. by J. H. Woods. Delhi: Motilal Banarsidass, 1966, first published by Harvard University Press, 1914; *Patañjali's Yoga Sūtras with the Commentary of Vyāsa and the Gloss of Vāchaspati Miśra*, trans. by Rāma Prasāda. Delhi: Oriental Books, 1978; *Yogasūtra of Patañjali with the Commentary of Vyāsa*, trans. by Bangali Baba. Delhi: Motilal Banarsidass, 1976.

3. *Pātañjala-Yogāsūtra-Bhāṣya Vivaraṇam* of Śaṅkara-Bhagavatpāda, edited by Polkam Sri Rama Sastri and S. R. Krishnamurthi Sastri. Madras: Government Oriental Manuscripts Library, 1952. For an English translation of Book I, see: *Śaṅkara on the Yoga-Sūtras*, translated by Trevor Leggett. London: Routledge and Kegan Paul, 1981. All four books have been translated and published by Kegan Paul International in 1990. There is debate among scholars over the authenticity of Śaṅkara's authorship. Legett, the translator, takes the text to be Śaṅkara's. W. Halbfass in *Tradition and Reflection* (Albany: State University of New York Press, 1991, pp. 205–242), gives a critical analysis of questions regarding Śaṅkara's authorship of the *Vivaraṇa* commentary. T. S. Rukmani, in her 1992 article, "The Problem of the Authorship of the Yogasutrabhāṣyavivaraṇa," *Journal of Indian Philosophy*, vol. 20, pp. 419–423, offers several reasons to question Śaṅkara's authorship. While the issue remains open, there seems to be a growing trend to accept the commentary as Śaṅkara's own, and this is the position I shall follow in this book.

4. Gerald Larson, "The Vedāntinization of Sāṁkhya," an unpublished lecture given at the Annual Meeting, American Academy of Religion, 1982.

5. Translation by Rama Prasāda (cited above in note 2), pp. 15–16.

6. Ibid., p. 156.

7. Ibid., pp. 17–18.

8. *Śaṅkara on the Yoga Sūtras*, trans. by Trevor Leggett, p. 49.

9. Translation by Rama Prasāda of *Yoga Sūtra* I:7, pp. 16–17.

10. Translation of J. H. Woods, p. 23.

11. Ibid.

12. *Śaṅkara on the Yoga Sūtras*, p. 50.

13. Swami Hariharānanda Āraṇya, *Yoga Philosophy of Patañjali*, trans. by P. N. Mukerji. Calcutta: University of Calcutta, 1977, p. 29.

14. See Vachaspati Miśra's gloss on *Yoga Sūtra* I:24.

15. *Śaṅkara on the Yoga Sūtras*, p. 89.

16. Vyāsa on I:25, as quoted in Śaṅkara's Vivaraṇa and translated by Trevor Leggett, p. 89.

17. Ibid., p. 94.

18. Ibid., p. 108.

19. See my survey of this viewpoint in *The Sphoṭa Theory of Language*. Delhi: Motilal Banarsidass, 1980, and in *The Philosophy of the Grammarians* by Harold Coward and K. Kunjunni Raja. Princeton: Princeton University Press, 1990.

20. Translation quoted is by Trevor Leggett, *Śaṅkara on the Yoga Sūtras*, p. 124.

21. Friedrich Heiler, *Prayer: A Study in the History of Psychology of Religion*. New York: Oxford University Press, 1958, p. 65.

22. M. Eliade, *Yoga: Immortality and Freedom*. Princeton: Princeton University Press, 1969, p. 75.

23. As an example, see *C. G. Jung Letters*, vol. 1. London: Routledge and Kegan Paul, 1973, p. 247.

24. Translation by Trevor Leggett, *Śaṅkara on the Yoga Sūtras*, p. 124.

25. Ibid., p. 125.

26. Ibid.

27. Ibid., p. 126.

28. The contention that "devotion to Īśvara was chosen by most of the yogis as their path to release" was stated to me by Professor T. R. V. Murti in my reading of this text with him.

29. M. Eliade, *Yoga: Immortality, and Freedom*, p. 74.

CHAPTER THREE
THE YOGA PSYCHOLOGY UNDERLYING BHARTṚHARI'S *VĀKYAPADĪYA*

1. For the Sāṅkhya school, see Vol. IV, Encyclopedia of Indian Philosophies, *Sāṁkhya*. G. Larson and R. S. Bhattacharya (eds.). Delhi: Motilal Banarsidass, 1987.

2. K. A. S. Iyer, *Bhartṛhari*. Poona: Deccan College, 1969.

3. Gaurinath Sastri, *The Philosophy of Word and Meaning*. Calcutta: Sanskrit College, 1959. See also Sastri's recent *The Philosophy of Bhartṛhari*. Delhi: Bharativa Vidya Prakashan, 1991.

4. Another contemporary scholar, K. Kunjunni Raja, recognizes the importance of the psychological side of Bhartṛhari's thought but analyzes it in terms of modern European associationalist psychology, a theory completely foreign to Bhartṛhari's thought and the thought forms of his day. See his *Indian Theories of Meaning*. Adyar: Adyar Library, 1963.

5. See Harold Coward and K. Kunjunni Raja, *The Philosophy of the Grammarians*. Princeton: Princeton University Press, 1990, pp. 44–50.

6. *Patañjali's Yoga Sūtras*, I:24–29.

7. Ibid., I:24–25.

8. Ibid., II:18, *bhāṣya*.

9. Ibid., I:26.

10. Ibid., I:25.

11. Ibid., I:24.

12. Iyer, *Bhartṛhari*, pp. 90–93. As Iyer has observed, this parallel was noticed by Helārāja, who quotes from Vyāsa's commentary on Yoga Sūtra I:25 in this context.

13. *Yoga Sūtras*, I:24, *ṭīkā*.

14. For the *Yoga Sūtras*, all experience of self-consciousness or thinking, this metaphysical assumption of wrong identification between *puruṣa* and *prakṛti* is held to obtain. Since our concern in this chapter is with the psychology of thinking and not the ultimate nature of the metaphysics involved, the discussion proceeds as if the *sattva* aspect of *prakṛti* were indeed real consciousness of illumination. This is in accord with the Yoga view of the nature of psychological processes at the thinking level. The *sattva* aspect of the thinking substance (*citta*), insofar as it is absolutely clear, takes on or reflects the intelligence (*cāitanya*) of *puruṣa*. For practical purposes, therefore, no duality appears, and *prakṛti* may be treated as self-illuminating (see *ṭīkā* [explanation] on *Yoga Sūtra* I:17).

15. S. N. Dasgupta finds that both the *Yoga Sūtras* and the *Vākyapadīya* adopt a kind of commonsense identification or ontological unity between the whole (the universal) and the parts (the particular manifestations). The three *guṇas* are the one universal genus, and it is the *guṇas* in various collocations that show themselves as the particular manifestations. *Yoga Philosophy*. Calcutta: University of Calcutta, 1930, pp. 120–26.

16. *Yoga Sūtras*, III:9.
17. Ibid., I:5.
18. Ibid., I:12.
19. Ibid., II:4–6.
20. Ibid., I:18, *ṭīkā*.
21. *Vākyapadīya*, *vṛtti* on I:51.
22. Ibid., *vṛtti* on I:1.
23. *Yoga Sūtras*, II:19, *bhāṣya*. Although for our present purpose, the inherent knowledge aspect of the *buddhittattva* is the point of focus, it should be realized that the *buddhittattva*, as the collective of all the individual minds (*buddhi*) with their beginningless *saṁskāras* of ignorance (*avidyā*) from previous births, also contains within it the inherent *avidyā* of the individual souls. And from the viewpoint of language, this *avidyā* would be composed of all the residual traces of the use of words in previous lives (*śabdabhāvanā*). See also Iyer, *Bhartṛhari*, p. 91.
24. S. N. Dasgupta, *The Study of Patañjali*. Calcutta: University of Calcutta, 1920, p. 53.
25. Iyer, *Bhartṛhari*, p. 149.
26. S. N. Dasgupta, *A History of Indian Philosophy*. Cambridge: The University Press, 1932, vol. I, p. 250.
27. Dasgupta, *Yoga Philosophy*, p. 209.
28. *Yoga Sūtras*, III:41.
29. *Vākyapadīya*, II:117–18 and I:122.
30. Ibid., I:46–47 and I:142.
31. Ibid., I:84, *vṛtti*.
32. *Yoga Sūtras*, *bhāṣya* on III:17. J. H. Woods translation.
33. Ibid., III:41, *ṭīkā*.
34. Ibid., III:17, *ṭīkā*. See also *Vākyapadīya* I:84.
35. Ibid., III:17, *bhāṣya*.
36. Iyer, *Bhartṛhari*, pp. 205–07 and 372. Bhartṛhari shows this superimposition to hold at all levels of linguistic complexity and offers the example of the appearance of the whole meaning in each part of the *dvandva* compound.
37. *Yoga Sūtras*, III:17, *bhāṣya*.
38. Ibid., *ṭīkā*.
39. Ibid., *bhāṣya*.
40. *Vākyapadīya*, II:73.
41. Ibid., I:142, *vṛtti*.
42. *Yoga Sūtras* I:44.
43. *Vākyapadīya*, I:153–55.
44. Ibid., I:131, *vṛtti*. It should be noted that while this interpretation is based on *Yoga Sūtras* I:12–16, only one aspect of Yoga *vairāgya* is represented: the turning away of the mind from all forms of worldly attachment. For Patañjali's Yoga at its ultimate level, *vairāgya* also involves the turning away of the mind from all forms of *vāk* so that the "seeded" or *samprajñāta samādhi* gives way to a "nonseeded" or "nonword" *asamprajñāta* state. (See *Yoga Sūtras* I:50–51 and II:15 ff.). For Bhartṛhari, since consciousness is shot through with *vāk*, *samādhi* in its highest elevations will always be "seeded" with Vedic word (see *Vākyapadīya* I:123).
45. *Vākyapadīya* II:28, *bhāṣya*.
46. Ibid., II:30, *bhāṣya*.
47. See Jacob Needleman, *The New Religions*. Richmond Hill: Simon and Schuster, 1972; William McNamara, *The Human Adventure: Contemplation for Everyman*. New York: Doubleday, 1974; and Matthew Fox, *Breakthrough: Meister Eckhart's Creation Spirituality in New Translation*. New York: Doubleday, 1991.

48. *Vākyapadīya*, I:14.
49. *Yoga Sūtras*, II:49–52.
50. Ibid., II:47, *bhāṣya* and *ṭīkā*, and II:48.
51. Ibid., II:50–53.
52. As quoted in Eliade, *Yoga: Immortality and Freedom*, pp. 55–56.
53. *Vākyapadīya*, I:131, *vṛtti.*
54. *Yoga Sūtras*, III:4.
55. Dasgupta, *Yoga Philosophy*, p. 335.
56. *Yoga-Sāra-Saṅgraha of Vijñana Bhikṣu*, translated by Ganganatha Jha. Madras: Theosophical Publishing House, 1932, p. 88.
57. *Yoga Sūtras*, III:2.
58. Ibid., III:3, *bhāṣya.*
59. Ibid., III:5.
60. Ibid., I:42–44.
61. Ibid., I:43, *ṭīkā.*
62. Ibid., I:44, *bhāṣya.*
63. *Vākyapadīya*, II:152.
64. Iyer, *Bhartṛhari*, p. 90.

CHAPTER FOUR YOGA IN THE *VAIRĀGYA-ŚATAKA* OF BHARTṚHARI

1. "Nītiśataka," *sloka* 2, translated by B. S. Miller in *Bhartṛhari: Poems.* New York: Columbia University Press, 1967.
2. M. R. Kale, *The Nīti and Vairāgya Śatakas of Bhartṛhari.* Delhi: Motilal Banarsidass, 1902.
3. D. D. Kosambi, "The Epigrams Attributed to Bhartṛhari," *Singhi Jain Series*, 23, 1948, and "On the Authorship of the Satakatrayī," *Journal of Oriental Research*, 15 Madras, 1946, pp. 64–77.
4. See K. A. S. Iyer's careful discussion of this problem in his *Bhartṛhari*, pp. 10–12. Although Iyer agrees with Kosambi that we cannot definitely know who the author of the *Śatakas* was, Iyer finds no evidence that contradicts the traditional identification of Bhartṛhari the poet with Bhartṛhari the grammarian.
5. Wm. Theodore de Bary, foreword to Miller, *Bhartṛhari: Poems.*
6. Miller, *Bhartṛhari: Poems*, introduction, p. xxvii.
7. *Patañjali's Yoga Sūtras*, II:3–9 with Vyāsa's *bhāṣya* and Vācaspati Miśra's *ṭīkā.*
8. Ibid., II:4.
9. Ibid., II:5.
10. References to the *Vairāgya-Śataka* are to the *sloka* numbering in the Advaita Ashrama edition, Calcutta, 1963. The translations are by B. S. Miller unless otherwise noted.
11. *Yoga Sūtras* II:6.
12. Ibid., II:7.
13. *Vairāgya-Śataka*, Advaita Ashrama commentary on *sloka* 17, p. 11.
14. *Yoga Sūtras* II:8.
15. W. B. Yeats, "Sailing to Byzantium," in *A Little Treasury of Modern Poetry*, edited by Oscar Williams. New York: Scribner's, 1952, p. 69.
16. *Vairāgya-Śataka*, *sloka* 9, p. 6.
17. *Yoga Sūtras* II:9.

18. Ibid., I:12, *bhāṣya*.
19. Ibid., I:15.
20. Ibid., II:28.
21. Ibid., II:29.
22. Ibid., II:30.
23. Ibid., II:35.
24. *Vairāgya-Śataka, sloka* 14, p. 9.
25. *Yoga Sūtras* II:32.
26. Ibid., II:32.
27. *Vairāgya-Śataka, sloka* 77, p. 44.
28. *Yoga Sūtras* II:32, *bhāṣya*.
29. *Vairāgya-Śataka, slokas* 83 and 84, p. 48.
30. *Yoga Sūtras* II:32.
31. *Vairāgya-Śataka, sloka* 82.
32. *Yoga Sūtras* II:34, *bhāṣya*.
33. Ibid., II:46.
34. *Vairāgya-Śataka, sloka* 85, p. 49.
35. Ibid., see, e.g. *slokas* 89, 95 and 100.
36. Ibid., *sloka* 63, p. 37.
37. *Yoga Sūtras* III:4.
38. Ibid., *bhāṣya* on III:3.
39. Ibid., I:44, *bhāṣya*.

CHAPTER FIVE
FREUD, JUNG, AND YOGA ON MEMORY

1. *Patañjaliyogadarsanam*. Varanasi: Bhāratāya Vidyā Prakāśana, 1963.

2. A basic work of Sigmund Freud, with reference to memory and motivation, is found in his seminal but little-known work, "Project for a Scientific Psychology," in *The Origins of Psychoanalysis*, M. Bonaparte, A. Freud, and E. Kris (eds.). London: Imago Pub. Co. Ltd., 1954, pp. 347–445.

3. The views of Carl Jung with regard to memory, motivation and the unconscious are found scattered throughout his *Collected Works* published by Princeton University Press. See especially Jung's notions of the Collective Unconscious, archetypes, and individuation or symbol formation. For a reliable concise presentation of Jung's thought, see *The Psychology of C. G. Jung* by Jolande Jacobi. New Haven, CT: Yale University Press, 1973.

4. *Yoga Sūtras*, II. 12–14 & IV. 7–9. The following is a summary of *karma* as found in these passages of the *Yoga Sūtras*:

> *Karma* has its origin in afflictions
>
> *kleśamūlaḥ karmāśayaḥ* (Sūtra II. 12)
>
> It ripens into life-states, life-experiences, and life-time, if the root exists.
>
> *sati mūle tadvipāko jātyāyyurbhogāḥ* (Sūtra II. 13)
>
> Those [life-states, etc.], as the fruit, are pleasant or unpleasant, because they are produced from virtuous or non-virtuous causes.
>
> *te hlādaparitāpaphalāḥ puṇyāpuṇyahetuvāt* (Sūtra II. 14)

To those who understand, all [of those] is indeed pain, because change, anxiety, .. are painful and (the life-states, etc.) obstruct the operations of virtuous qualities.

In *Yoga Sūtra*, *karma* is equal to *vāsanā*.

pariṇāmatapasaṁskāraduḥkhair guṇavṛttivirodhāc ca duḥkham eva sarvaṁ vivekinaḥ (Sūtra II. 15)

A Yogin's *karma* is neither white nor black, for [all] others, it is threefold.

karmāsuklākṛṣnaṁ yoginas trividham itareṣām (Sūtra IV. 7)

From the [threefold *karma*] there come the impressions (*vāsanā*) of only those which are capable of bringing about their fruition. In *Yoga Sūtra*, *smṛti* is equal to *saṁskāra*.

tatas tadvipākānuguṇānām ekāb-hivyaktir vāsanānām (Sūtra IV. 8)

[The process of impression] continues uninterruptedly, even though there is a time lapse between births, places, and time, because memory and memory traces are of one substance.

jātideśakālavyavahitānām apy ānantaryaṁ smṛtisaṁskārayor ekarūpatvāt (Sūtra IV. 9)

Commentary on Sūtra IV. 9 states: *kutaś ca smṛtisaṁskārayor ekarūpatvāt/yathānubhavās tathā aṁskārāḥ te ca karmavāsanārūpāh/yathā ca vāsanās tathā smṛtir iti/jātideśakālavyavahitebhyaḥ saṁskārebhyaḥ smṛtiḥ smṛtiś ca punaḥ saṁskārā ity evam ete smṛtisaṃskārāḥ karmāśayavṛttilābhavaśāveśād abhivayajyante/. . . /vāsanāh saṁskārā āśayā ity arthaḥ/*

(Note: here, *saṁskāra* is better translated "memory traces," because unlike Sutra II. 15, *saṁskāra* is equated to *smṛti*.)

Therefore, according to this:

smṛti—saṁskāra—smṛti; the continuation of which is supported by *karma* (*karmābhivyañjakaṁ*) and *vāsanā* functions as the support for *saṁskāra* (memory traces) which produce *smṛti* (memory).

I acknowledge the assistance of my colleague Dr. L. S. Kawamura in interpreting these passages.

5. Gordon W. Allport, *Becoming*. New Haven, Connecticut: Yale University Press, 1955, pp. 7–17.

6. Edwin G. Boring, *A History of Experimental Psychology*, 2nd ed. New York: Appleton-Century-Crofts, 1950, p. 566.

7. Ibid., 702.

8. K. H. Pribram, "The Foundation of Psychoanalytic Theory: Freud's Neuropsychological Model," published for the first time in *Brain and Behaviour* 4, R. H. Pribram (ed.). Penguin Books, 1969, pp. 395–432.

9. Sigmund Freud, "Project for a Scientific Psychology," in *The Origins of Psychoanalysis*, M. Bonaparte, A. Freud, and E. Kris (eds.). London: Imago Pub. Co., 1954, pp. 347–445.

10. Surendranath Dasgupta, *Yoga as Philosophy and Religion*. Port Washington, NY: Kennikat Press, 1970, p. 177.

11. K. Pribram, "Foundation of Psychoanalytic Theory," p. 400.

12. Ibid.

13. John C. Eccles, "Conscious Memory: The Cerebral Processes Concerned in Storage and Retrieval," in *The Self and Its Brain*, by Karl R. Popper and John C. Eccles. London: Springer International, 1977, p. 377.

14. Ibid., p. 383.

15. Frances Crick and Christof Koch, "Towards a Neurobiological Theory of Consciousness" in *The Nature of Consciousness* Ned Block, Owen Flanagan and Gwen Guzeldere (eds.). Cambridge, Mass.: M.I.T. Press, 1997, pp. 284–85. The recent *Oxford Handbook of Memory* E. Tulving and F. Craik (eds.). Oxford: Oxford University Press, 2000, also shows that this thinking is still very current.

16. "Conscious Memory," op. cit., p. 385.

17. *Yoga Sūtra* II:15.

18. An article by Bernard Baars reviews recent research suggesting that conscious experience involves a selective choice and constructive act of memory and perception inputs. "Contrastive Phenomenology," in *The Nature of Consciousness*, op. cit., pp. 188–89.

19. Freud's theory as summarized by K. Pribram, "Foundations of Psychoanalytic Theory," pp. 400–401.

20. K. Pribram, "Foundations of Psychoanalytic Theory," p. 401.

21. Calvin S. Hall, *A Primer of Freudian Psychology*. New York: Mentor Books, 1958, p. 24.

22. Op. cit., p. 25.

23. Op. cit., p. 86.

24. Sigmund Freud, "Unconscious Motivation in Everyday Life," in *Studies in Motivation*, David C. McClelland (ed.). New York: Appleton-Century-Crofts, 1955, pp. 3–18.

25. Ibid., p. 16.

26. *Yoga Sūtras* I. 5 and II. 4.

27. *Yoga Sūtras* I. 51 and III. 5.

28. From Oct. 1938 to June 1939, Jung lectured on "The Process of Individuation" at the Eidgenössische Technische Hochschule, Zürich (E. T. H. Lectures). Unpublished notes show that during the summer of 1939, Jung's lectures IV., V., and VI. dealt in detail with Patañjali's *Yoga Sūtras*.

29. C. G. Jung, *Memories, Dreams, Reflections*. Aniela Jaffe (ed.). New York: Vintage Books, 1965. See pp. 170–99 and especially p. 197.

30. For a detailed analysis of the influence of Yoga on Jungian psychology, see H. G. Coward, "Jung's Encounter with Yoga," *The Journal of Analytical Psychology* 23, no. 4, 1978, pp. 339–57.

31. *C. G. Jung: Letters*, vol. I, G. Adler and A. Jaffe (eds.). London: Routledge and Kegan Paul, 1973, pp. 263–64.

32. C. G. Jung, *On the Nature of the Psyche, Collected Works*, vol. 8, p. 349.

33. Jolande Jacobi, *The Psychology of C. G. Jung*. New Haven, CT: Yale University Press, 1973, p. 34.

34. *C. G. Jung: Letters*, vol. I, p. 226n. In this note Adler is quoting from Jung's "A Psychological Approach to the Dogma of the Trinity." *Collected Works*, 11, par. 222.

35. Ibid., pp. 35–36. See also Jung's *Collected Works*, 11, pp. 518–19.

36. Ibid., pp. 30–33.

37. C. G. Jung, *On the Tibetan Book of the Dead, Collected Works*, 11, p. 517.

38. Ibid., p. 517.

39. Eido Roshi, "Zen Mystical Practice," in *Mystics and Scholars: The Calgary Conference on Mysticism*, 1976, Harold Coward and Terence Penelhum (eds.). Waterloo, Ontario, Canada: Wilfrid Laurier University Press, 1977, pp. 27–29.

40. *Yoga Sūtras* III. 9 and IV. 27.

41. *Yoga Sūtras* IV. 28 and 29.

42. C. G. Jung, *E. T. H. Lectures*, p. 11.

43. C. G. Jung, *The Structure and Dynamics of the Psyche, Collected Works*. 8, p. 390.

44. See the review article by R. C. Bolles, "Cognition and Motivation: Some Historical Trends," in *Cognitive Views of Human Motivation*, Bernard Weiner (ed.). New York: Academic Press, 1974, pp. 1–20, as well as current discussions of memory and consciousness in the authoritative collections of recent research, *The Nature of Consciousness* (1997), op. cit. and *The Oxford Handbook of Memory* (2000), op. cit.

CHAPTER SIX
WHERE JUNG DRAWS THE LINE IN HIS ACCEPTANCE OF PATAÑJALI'S YOGA

1. See Jung's biography, *Memories, Dreams, Reflections*, Aniela Jaffé (ed.). New York: Vintage Books, 1965.

2. See Curtis D. Smith, *Jung's Quest for Wholeness*. Albany: State University of New York Press, 1990.

3. C. G. Jung, *Collected Works*, Vol. II. Princeton: Princeton University Press, 1969, p. 505 (hereafter referred to as *C. W.*).

4. C. G. Jung, "The Holy Men of India," *C. W.* 11, p. 580.

5. *C. G. Jung: Letters*, Vol. II, Gerhard Adler (ed.). Princeton: Princeton University Press, 1974, p. 438.

6. Ibid. Within Western psychology, Jung is criticized as falling into the same trap of neglecting the body and the psycho-physiological reality in his psychology. See Edward Whitmont, "Prefatory Remarks to Jung's 'Reply to Buber,'" *Spring*, 1973, p. 193.

7. Ibid.

8. Ibid., pp. 234–35. See also F. X. Charet, Spiritualism and the Foundations of C. G. Jung's Psychology. Albany: State University of New York Press, 1993.

9. *Memories, Dreams, Reflections*, op. cit., pp. 200–23. See also *C. G. Jung: Letters*, Vol. I, pp. 261–64.

10. Gilbert Ryle, *The Concept of Mind*. New York: Penguin, 1963, pp. 301–11.

11. Ibid., p. 307.

12. Ibid., p. 308.

13. C. G. Jung, "On the Nature of the Psyche," *C. W.* 8, pp. 171–73. Here Jung seems to echo William James's notion of a flimsy threshold separating the differing energy levels of the conscious and the unconscious. See James's *Varieties of Religious Experience*. New York: Mentor, 1958.

14. "The Process of Individuation: Notes on Lectures given at the Eidgenössische Technische Hochschule, Zürich by Prof. C. G. Jung, October 1938–June 1939." E. T. H. Lectures recorded by Barbara Hannah. Unpublished manuscript.

15. Ibid., pp. 1–10, 42.

16. C. G. Jung, "On the Secret of the Golden Flower," *C. W.* 13, p. 14.

17. C. G. Jung, "The Structure and Dynamics of the Psyche," *C. W.* 8, p. 390.

18. *C. G. Jung: Letters*, Vol. I, op. cit., pp. 262–64.

19. Ibid., p. 264.

20. *Yoga Sūtras*, op. cit., III:34–35.

21. Jadunath Sinha, *Indian Psychology: Cognition*. Calcutta: Sinha Publishing House, 1958, p. 334. Of the schools of Indian philosophy, only the materialist Cārvāka, the Mīmāṁsaka, and the Viśiṣṭādvaita Vedānta reject the two-level theory of perception and accept only ordinary sense perception as a valid source of knowledge. The Sāṅkhya-Yoga, Nyāya-Vaiśeṣika, Advaita Vedānta, Grammarian, Buddhist, and Jaina schools all accept supersensuous

perceptions (*pratibhā*), although they give different accounts of them. For an excellent account of these various views of *pratibhā*, see Gopinath Kaviraj, "The Doctrine of Pratibhā in Indian Philosophy," *Annals of the Bhandarkar Oriental Research Institute*, 1924, pp. 1–18, 113–32.

22. *Yoga Sūtras*, op. cit., I:43.
23. Ibid., I:44.
24. Ibid., III:32.
25. C. G. Jung, "On the Tibetan Book of the Great Liberation," *C. W.* 11, p. 504.
26. Ibid., p. 505.
27. *C. G. Jung: Letters*, vol. I, op. cit., p. 175.
28. C. G. Jung, "The Archetypes and the Collective Unconscious," *C. W.* 9, pt. I, p. 282.
29. C. G. Jung, "The Structure and Dynamics of the Psyche," *C. W.* 8, pp. 140–41.
30. Ibid., p. 141.
31. *The Psychology of C. G. Jung*, op. cit., p. 12.
32. Richard Evans, *Conversations with Carl Jung*. New York: Van Nostrand, 1964, p. 74.
33. *The Psychology of C. G. Jung*, op. cit., pp. 32–33.
34. C. G. Jung, Foreword to "Introduction to Zen Buddhism," *C. W.* 11, p. 550.
35. Ibid., pp. 551–57.
36. *C. G. Jung: Letters*, Vol. II, op. cit., p. 223.
37. Ibid.
38. *C. G. Jung: Letters*, Vol. I, op. cit., pp. 389–90.
39. *Indian Psychology: Cognition*, op. cit., p. 339.
40. "The Doctrine of Pratibhā in Indian Philosophy," op. cit., p. 2.
41. *Yoga Sūtras*, I:48.
42. "The Doctrine of Pratibhā in Indian Philosophy," op. cit., p. 9.
43. E. T. H. Lectures, op. cit., p. 136.
44. "On the Secret of the Golden Flower," *C. W.* 13, p. 8.
45. *Memories, Dreams, Reflections*, op. cit., p. 393.
46. C. G. Jung, "Conscious, Unconscious, and Individuation," in "The Archetypes and the Collective Unconscious," *C. W.* 9, pt. I, pp. 275f.
47. "The Structure and Dynamics of the Psyche," *C. W.* 8, p. 226.
48. "Two Essays on Analytical Psychology," *C. W.* 7, para. 274. See also "The Psychology of Transference," in "The Practice of Psychotherapy," *C. W.* 16, para. 536. See also Sean Kelly, *Individuation and the Absolute*. New York: Paulist Press, 1993, p. 28.

CHAPTER SEVEN
MYSTICISM IN JUNG AND PATAÑJALI'S YOGA

1. Walter H. Principe, "Mysticism: Its Meaning and Varieties," in *Mystics and Scholars*, Harold Coward and Terence Penelhum (eds.). Waterloo: Wilfrid Laurier University Press, 1976, p.1.
2. W. T. Stace, *Mysticism and Philosophy*. London: Macmillan, 1961, p. 15.
3. Ibid., pp. 13–18.
4. Rudolf Otto, *The Idea of the Holy*. New York: Oxford University Press 1963, p. 113.
5. Frederick C. Copleston, *Religion and Philosophy*. Dublin: Gill and Macmillan, 1974, p. 90.
6. William James, *The Varieties of Religious Experience*. New York: Mentor 1958, pp. 58ff.

7. *Spiritual presence* is Arnold Toynbee's term which Walter Stace adopted in his *Mysticism and Philosophy*, op. cit., p. 5.

8. *The Idea of the Holy*, op. cit., p. 7.

9. *Absolute* is the term adopted by Evelyn Underhill in her *Mysticism*. New York: Meridan, 1955. See also Steven T. Katz (ed.), *Mysticism and Religious Traditions*, Oxford: Oxford University Press, 1983, for an analysis of how this "Absolute" has been experienced by mystics of various religious traditions.

10. *Religion and Philosophy*, op. cit., p. 75.

11. Ibid.

12. *The Varieties of Religious Experience*, op. cit., pp. 385–86.

13. C. G. Jung, *Memories, Dreams, Reflections*. New York: Vintage, 1965, Cp. XII.

14. BBC Interview of C. G. Jung by Laurens van der Post. "The Story of Carl Gustav Jung—Mystery that Heals," BBC-TV, 1972.

15. *Memories, Dreams, Reflections*, p. 338.

16. *Memories, Dreams, Reflections*, op. cit., p. 336.

17. Ibid., p. 337.

18. Ibid., p. 338.

19. C. G. Jung, "The Holy Men of India" in *C. W.* 11:576–86.

20. Ibid., p. 581.

21. C. G. Jung, "The Process of Individuation in the Exercitia spiritulia of St. Ignatius of Loyola," June 1939–March 1940, unpublished Eidgenössische Technische Hochschule Lectures, Zurich (E. T. H. Lectures), pp. 122–23.

22. Ibid., p. 123.

23. It is of interest to note in passing that after some decades of neglect, modern Western psychology in the 1990s returned to a serious examination of consciousness as perhaps the most foundational concept to be understood, thus opening the way for new dialogue with both Jung and Yoga. See *The Nature of Consciousness*, Ned Block, Owen Flanagan, and Gwen Guzeldere (eds.). Cambridge: M.I.T. Press, 1997.

24. C. G. Jung, "Psychology and Religion," *C. W.* 11:23ff.

25. For more on Jung's understanding of synchronicity in religious experience, see Harold Coward, "Taoism and Jung: Synchronicity and the Self," *Philosophy East and West*, Vol. 46, 1996, pp. 477–96. See also Robert Aziz, *C. G. Jung's Psychology of Religion and Synchronicity*. Albany: State University of New York Press, 1990.

26. C. G. Jung, "Concerning Mandala Symbolism," *C. W.* 9, Pt. 1:357.

27. Another image which Jung sometimes used in the same way as the *maṇḍala* was that of the tree. This is especially seen in his 1945 Festschrift article, "The Philosophical Tree," written in honor of Gustav Senn, Professor of Botany, University of Basel. In it Jung says, "If a mandala may be described as a symbol of the self seen in cross section, then the tree would represent a profile view of it: the self depicted as a process of growth." *C. W.* 13, p. 253.

28. C. G. Jung, "Psychology and Religion," *C. W.* 11:79–80.

29. C. G. Jung, "Commentary on The Secret of the Golden Flower," *C. W.* 13:26–28.

30. W. T. Stace, *The Teachings of the Mystics* (New York: Mentor, 1960), pp. 14–15.

31. C. G. Jung, "The Psychology of Eastern Meditation," *C. W.* 11:574–75.

32. C. G. Jung, "The Holy Men of India," *C. W.* 11:584.

33. The following section is an interpretation of Patañjali's *Yoga Sūtras*, especially *sūtras* 1:41–51, with the Commentary (*Bhāsya*) by Vyāsa and the Gloss (*Tika*) by Vācaspati Miśra. *Patañjali-Yogadarsanam*. Varanasi: Bhārātīya Vidhyā Prakāśana, 1963. The best English translation is by Rama Prasada, Allahabad: Bhuvaneswari Asrama, 1924.

34. See *Sāṅkhya Kārikā of Īśvara Krishna*, Trans. by J. Davies. Calcutta: Susil Gupta, 1947.

35. *Yoga Sūtra* 11:18, *bhāṣya.*

36. See Gopinath Kaviraj, "The Doctrine of Pratibhā in Indian Philosophy," *Annals of the Bhandarkar Oriental Research Institute* (1924):1–18 and 113–32.

37. *Yoga Sūtra* 1:41.

38. Ibid., *bhāṣya.*

39. This is the "seedless" or "objectless" *samādhi* described by Patañjali in *Yoga Sūtra* 1:51.

40. *Yoga Sūtra* 1:42, *bhāsya.*

41. Ibid.

42. Ibid., *ṭikā.*

43. *Yoga Sūtra* 1:43, *bhāsya.*

44. *Amos* 6:1–14.

45. *John* 4:1–26.

46. *Yoga Sūtra* 1:43, *ṭikā*. See also Christopher Chapple, "The Unseen Seer and the Field: Consciousness in Samkhya and Yoga," in *The Problem of Pure Consciousness: Mysticism and Philosophy*, Robert K. C. Forman (ed.). Oxford: Oxford University Press, 1990, pp. 66–69.

47. *Yoga Sūtra* 1:51, *bhāsya.*

48. Chapter III:45 of the *Yoga Sūtras* gives a complete list of the psychic powers and how to attain them. See Ian Whicher, *The Integrity of the Yoga Darśana*. Albany: State University of New York Press, 1998, p. 112, for a description and discussion of the *siddhis.*

CHAPTER EIGHT
THE LIMITS OF HUMAN NATURE IN YOGA AND TRANSPERSONAL PSYCHOLOGY

1. For a good overview of Western thought in this regard, see John Passmore, *The Perfectibility of Man*. New York: Charles Scribner's Sons, 1970.

2. Jean Varenne, *Yoga and the Hindu Tradition.* Delhi: Motilal Banarsidass, 1989.

3. Mircea Eliade, *Yoga: Immortality and Freedom*. Translated from the French by Willard R. Trask. Princeton: Princeton University Press, 1969, p. 363.

4. Andrew O. Fort and Patricia Y. Mumme (eds.), *Living Liberation in Hindu Thought.* Albany: State University of New York Press, 1996, p. 1. See also Andrew O. Fort (ed.) *Jīvanmukti in Transformation: Embodied Liberation in Advaita and Neo-Vedanta.* Albany: State University of New York Press, 1998. See also the "Feature Review" of the Fort and Mumme volume by Arvind Sharma in *Philosophy East and West*, Vol. 48, 1998, pp. 142–61.

5. *Living Liberation in Hindu Thought*, op. cit., p. 1.

6. *Jīvan-Mukti-Viveka of Swami Vidāraṇya*, Trans. by Swami Moksadananda. Calcutta: Advaita Ashrama, 1996.

7. Patricia Y. Mumme, "Living Liberation in a Comparative Perspective," in *Living Liberation in Hindu Thought*, op. cit., p. 247.

8. See Andrew O. Fort, *Jīvanmukti in Transformation.* Albany: State University of New York Press, 1998.

9. See chapter 10, "A Liberated Being Being Liberated: The Case of Ramana Maharshi," *Jīvanmukti in Transformation*, op. cit., pp. 134–51.

10. *Yoga Sūtra* II:2, *Bhāsya.*

11. Christopher Key Chapple, "Living Liberation in Sāṃkhya and Yoga," in *Living Liberation in Hindu Thought*, op. cit., p. 124.

12. *Yoga Sūtras* I:42–44.

13. Andrew O. Fort, *The Self and Its States.* Delhi: Motilal Banarsidass, 1990, p. 116.

14. Michael Washburn, *The Ego and the Dynamic Ground.* Albany: State University of New York Press, 1988.

15. Ibid., p. v.

16. Ibid., p. 20.

17. Alan Roland, *In Search of Self in India and Japan: Toward a Cross-Cultural Psychology.* Princeton: Princeton University Press, 1988.

18. Ibid., p. 10.

19. Charles Tart (ed.), *Transpersonal Psychologies.* New York: Harper Colophon, 1975.

20. Ibid., p. 2.

21. Robert Ornstein (ed.), *The Nature of Human Consciousness: A Book of Readings.* San Francisco: W. H. Freeman, 1973, p. xi.

22. In Tart, op. cit., p. 244.

23. Ibid., p. 262.

24. John Hick, *The Fifth Dimension: An Exploration of the Spiritual Realm.* Oxford: Oneworld, 1999, p. 141. Hick does allow, following Kant's lead, that human individuality, having served its purpose, may one day be transcended, but that such a final state must be "far beyond this life." (p. 136) This claim imposes a Western Christian Kantian presupposition as to what is possible for human nature and is the basis for Hick's epistemological conclusion that claims of literal unity, such as Yoga makes of experience in this life, must be "metaphorical" rather than "literal." Hick's conclusions may be right if the presuppositions upon which he bases them happen to be right. But we currently have no philosophical helicopter that will take us to a no-presupposition place from which we can evenhandedly judge between the very different presuppositions of, say, Kant and Patañjali so as to determine that one had it right and the other had it wrong, or both, or neither. Thus my counsel for a critical openmindedness to the study of all claims as to the possibilities of human nature.

25. *Yoga Sūtras,* op. cit., IV:25, *Ṭika* of Vachaspati Mishra, as translated by J. H. Woods, in *The Yoga System of Patañjali.* Delhi: Motilal Banarsidass, 1966, p. 338.

glossary of sanskrit terms

abhiniveśa. Clinging to life.

abhyāsa. Habitual steadying of the mind in Yogic concentration.

adhyāsa. Superimposition.

āgama. Scriptural truth, including *śruti, smṛti,* the epics and Purāṇas.

ahaṁkāra. Ego.

ahiṃsā. Nonviolence in thought and deed.

akliṣṭa. Unafflicted, pure, free from ignorance.

antaḥkaraṇa. The internal mental organ composed of the *buddhi, ahaṃkāra,* and *manas* functions.

anumāna. Inference.

aparigraha. Absence of avarice.

apauruṣeya. Used to indicate that Vedic scripture is authorless, eternal, and therefore safeguarded from error.

artha. Word-meaning as distinct from word-sound; the inner meaning of a word; object.

āsana. Yogic posture for the purpose of immobilizing the body, e.g., lotus position.

asmitā. Egoity.

asteya. Nonstealing.

ātman. Self or soul.

AUM. The sacred syllable of Hinduism that symbolizes and evokes all levels of consciousness, all knowledge of the Divine.

avidyā. The obscuring veil of human ignorance that, when removed, reveals knowledge of reality.

bhāṣya. Commentary.

bīja. Seed or seed state.

brahmacarya. Celibacy in thought and action.

Brahman. The Absolute; the Divine; sometimes characterized as pure consciousness.

buddhi. The level of consciousness characterized by intelligent discrimination; intellect.

buddhitattva. Pure collective or universal consciousness containing within it all intellects of individuals.

citta. Consciousness, including both the level of awareness and the level of unconsciousness.

citta vṛtti. A particular mental state.

darśana. Viewpoint; philosophical school.

dhāraṇā. Short Yogic concentration with momentary loss of subject-object duality.

dharma. One's religious and moral duty in life; doing one's *dharma* produces spiritual merit; also may mean truth.

dhvani. The physical sound or the uttered syllables of a word.

dhvani. In Indian aesthetics, the use of poetic or dramatic words to suggest or evoke a feeling that is too deep, intense, and universal to be spoken.

dhyāna. Yogic concentration lasting several *dhṇraṇs*; the uninterrupted flow of fixed concentration upon an *artha*, or object.

dveṣa. Disgust.

guṇa. A characteristic or quality; usually refers to the three *guṇas* of consciousness: *sattva, rajas,* and *tamas.*

guru. Spiritual teacher.

Īśvara. In the Yoga view, the divine *guru* of the ancient *ṛṣis*; the Divine Word of the scripture in its transcendental essence that makes up the pure consciousness of Īśvara.

Īśvarapranidhana. Offering up of all action and thought to the Lord (Īśvara).

jīva. The empirical self, individual being.

jñāna. True, unobscured knowledge of the word or object.

kaivalya. The Saṅkhya term for release; the *puruṣa* fully revealed in its isolated splendor.

kārikā. A concise verse requiring an interpretative commentary for its understanding.

karma. The trace or seed left behind by each thought or action that predisposes one to a similar thought or action in the future.

kleśas. Constantly changing painful states of consciousness.

kliṣṭa. Afflicted by ignorance.

kratu. An energy (within the word) that seeks to burst forth into expression; the drive to diversity within the unitary whole, or *sphoṭa.*

madhyamā vāk. Language as thought that has not yet been uttered.

mahāvākyas. The great criterion sentences of the Upaniṣads, e.g., "That thou art."

manas. The mental organ that collects and coordinates information.

mantra. A verse of poetic scripture in praise of the Divine.

Mīmāṁsā. One of the six orthodox schools of Indian philosophy; argues for the authorlessness and eternality of the letter sounds of the Vedas.

mokṣa. Release, freedom from the suffering and bondage of this world, oneness with the Divine.

nāda. Physical sound.

nirvāṇa. State of release or enlightenment.

nirvicāra. A pure form of *samādhi* in which the meaning or object is fully revealed in its very essence; no notions of time, space or causality are present.

nirvitarka. Trance concentration upon the gross form of the object, but freed from the confusion of memory and the conventional use of words.

niyamas. Positive Yogic practices for the purifying of body and mind.

paśyantī vāk. Level of intuitive or flashlike understanding of the sentence meaning as a whole.

prajñā. Direct intuitive knowledge of things as they are in themselves, rather than as they appear to us.

prakṛti. Nonintelligent matter, one side of the Sāṅkhya-Yoga metaphysical duality.

pramā. True cognition or knowing, as distinct from false knowing.

pramāṇa. A true or valid way of knowing, e.g., perception; although there is argument in Indian philosophy, six *pramāṇas* are often discussed: perception, inference, analogy, presumption, nonapprehension (*abhāva*), and the revelatory power of speech (*śabda*); it is with the *pramāṇa* of *śabda* that Bhartṛhari is most concerned.

prāṇa. Breath; the instrumental cause of speech at the lower levels of language.

praṇava. AUM, the sacred "root" sound from which all language flows forth.

prāṇāyāma. Regulation of respiration.

pratibhā. Immediate supersensuous intuition; supernormal perception that transcends the ordinary categories of time, space, and causality and has the capacity to directly "grasp" the real nature of things.

pratyāhāra. Withdrawal of senses from worldly attachments.

pratyaya. Ground or support in which the word-sound and word-meaning inhere.

puruṣa. An individual pure consciousness, one side of the Sāṅkhya-Yoga metaphysical duality.

rāga. Passion.

rajas. The aspect of consciousness that is passion or energy.

rasa. A dominant mood evoked in the aesthetic experience of poetry and drama.

rasadhvani. The inner essence of the aesthetic experience that is beyond all conceptual expression.

rīti. Poetic style.

ṛṣi. An original seer or "speaker" of Hindu scripture. One who has purged himself of all ignorance, rendering his consciousness transparent to the Divine Word.

śabda. Word or words that when spoken convey knowledge, especially of the Divine.

Śabdabrahman. The Absolute, the Divine for Bhartṛhari; the intertwined unity of word and consciousness that is the one ultimate reality; for Bhartṛhari both the material and efficient cause of creation; also called the Divine Word, or *Daivī-Vāk.*

śabdapūrvayoga. The spiritual discipline of meditating upon the Divine Word, leads to *mokṣa,* or release.

Śabdatattva. Brahman as the omniscient word-principle.

sādhana. A personal discipline or practice for spiritual self-realization.

samādhi. Trance state of consciousness with no subject-object distinction.

samprajñāta samādhi. "Seeded" or trance concentration upon an object, as opposed to "unseeded" or trance concentration without an object.

saṁsāra. Rebirth in the suffering and bondage of this world; the continual round of birth-death-rebirth; the world of phenomena.

saṁskāra. A memory trace that has the dynamic quality of a seed that is constantly ready to sprout.

saṃtoṣa. Contentment.

saṅketa. Convention of language usage as maintained by the elders in this and previous generations.

Sāṅkhya. One of the six orthodox schools of Indian philosophy; argues for a dualism of matter (*prakṛti*) and individual souls (*puruṣas*).

śānta rasa. The aesthetic experience of spiritual serenity; the absolute *rasa* into which all other emotions subside.

śāstra. Authoritative teaching.

sattva. The aspect of consciousness that is brightness or intelligence.

sattva saṁskāra. Series, continuous flow of pure consciousness as it would be in the mind of the Lord (Īśvara); no distinction between word and meaning, but only the constant presence of meaning as a whole.

satyā. Truthfulness.

savicāra. A form of *samādhi* in which little error is present; the intensity of concentration produces transparent *sattva* so that the true meaning or object (*artha*) stands revealed with only slight distortions of time, space, and causality.

savitarka. Indistinct Yogic concentration or *samādhi* in which memory, word, and object are indiscriminately mixed together.

sāyuja. The highest spiritual goal of union with the Divine.

svādhāya. Concentrated scriptural study, including both meditation upon verses and chanting of AUM.

svarga. "Heaven," not the final release or goal of Hinduism, but the place where the fruits of the spiritual merit one has achieved are enjoyed.

tamas. The aspect of consciousness that is dullness or inertia.

tanmātras. Subtle primary elements; inner counterparts to the gross sense experiences of sound, touch, color, shape, flavor, and smell.

tapas. Psychic heat or energy generated from the practice of austerities; bearing with equanimity the pairs of opposites such as heat and cold, hunger and thirst.

vāgyoga. Yoga or concentration upon speech.

vaikharī vāk. Gross or physical level of uttered speech.

vairāgya. Turning away of the mind from all forms of worldly attachment.

vāk. Language that is thought of as having various levels, from the gross form of the spoken word to the subtle form of the highest intuition.

vākya sphoṭa. Intuitive understanding or direct perception of the sentence meaning as a whole idea.

varṇa. Letter sounds.

vāsanā. A habit pattern of thought and/or action, composed of reinforced *karmas.*

Vedānta. One of the six orthodox schools of Indian philosophy, often identified with the monistic absolutism of Śaṅkara.

Veda. The primary Hindu scriptures, including the early hymns (Saṃhitā), the Brāhmaṇas, Āranyakas, and Upaniṣads; the Saṃhitā are organized into four collections called *Ṛg*, *Sāma*, *Yajur*, and *Atharva*.

vikalpa. The mixing or superimposing of two or more mental states so that knowledge is obscured and error produced.

vṛtti. A commentary.

Vyākaraṇa. Grammar; one of the traditional schools of Indian philosophy; Patañjali and Bhartṛhari are among the leaders of this school.

yamas. Yogic practices of self-restraint, e.g., *ahiṃṣā*, or nonviolence.

Yoga. One of the six schools of orthodox Indian philosophy; describes a practical psychological discipline for achieving release, systematized by Patañjali.

yogāṅga. Steps or aids to the practice of Yoga.

index

active imagination, 64, 86
Adler, Gerhard, 57
Advaita Vedanta, 14, 16, 84, 85
āgama (verbal communication), 11ff., 17, 20, 23
archetype, 57, 58, 59, 60, 66, 68, 75
  God archetype, 73–77, 86
Aristotle, 11
āsana, 37, 39, 47
Ātman, 16, 48
AUM, 17, 18, 19, 20, 23, 36, 78, 91
Aurobindo, Sri, 84
avidyā, 24, 25, 28, 32, 33, 43, 44, 95

Bhaṛthari, 17, 21, 24, 41, 91, 95
  as poet, 41ff.
  on hearing, 30–35
  on speaking, 26–30
  Vairāgya-Śataka, 41–48
  Vākyapadīya, 21–40
Bhiksu, Vijñāna, 38
Brahman, 2, 16, 18, 23, 25, 82
Buddha, 6, 64, 77, 82, 92
Buddhist thought, 14, 77

Chapple, Christopher, 85
Chaudhuri, Haridas, 88
Christ, 74, 75, 76, 77, 81, 82
Christianity, 83, 86, 88
collective consciousness (*buddhitattva*), 27, 28, 29, 32
collective unconscious, 57, 58, 75
consciousness, 28, 29, 39, 43, 45, 48, 66, 68, 78, 83, 101
Copleston, Fredrick, 72
Crick, Francis, 54

Dasgupta, 27–28, 31, 95
dhāraṇā, 38, 39, 48
dharma, 16, 39
dhvani, 29, 30, 31, 32, 34, 39, 42
dhyāna, 38, 39, 48
dreams, 76

Eccles, Sir John, 53, 59, 91
ego, 2, 27, 28, 29, 34, 43, 58, 59, 60, 64, 65, 66, 67, 68, 69, 73, 74, 75, 76, 77, 81, 82, 84, 85, 86, 87
Eliade, Mircea, 1, 18, 20, 38, 83, 84
Evans-Wentz, W. Y., 56, 64

Fort, Andrew, 84, 85
freedom of choice, 53, 55, 56, 60, 91
Freud, S., 2, 7, 52, 53, 54, 55, 56, 57, 59, 62, 86, 91, 92, 98

God, 73, 74, 75, 77, 81
guru, 3, 4, 78, 84, 92

hearing, 30–40
Hick, John, 7, 89, 92, 105
Hubbard, A.M., 67
human nature, 2, 4, 7, 83–90, 91
  perfectability of, 85

idea, 26, 34
individuation, 69, 86, 100
inference, 12
intuition, 65
Īśvara, 12–20, 22, 23, 24, 25, 26, 35
I-tsing, 21, 41
Iyer, K. A. S., 22

James, William, 82
jīvan-mukti (living liberation), 84, 85, 92
Jīvan-Mukti-Viveka of Vidyaranya, 84
jñāna, 34, 79
Jung, Carl, 4, 6, 19, 56, 74, 79, 82, 83, 86, 89, 90, 91, 92, 98
  acceptance of Patañjali's Yoga, 61–69
  and *Karma*, 56–60
  and memory, 56–60, 63–64
  and mysticism, 73–77
  and perception, 65–67
  The Holy Men of India, 74

Kale, M. R., 41
Kant, I., 83
karma, 1, 3, 15, 16, 23, 47, 51, 52, 53, 54, 56, 59, 84, 91, 98–99
  Karma-saṁsāra, 19
knowledge, 67–69, 73
Kosambi, D. D., 41

language, 11ff., 23
  power of ordinary words, 12–14
  power of scriptural words, 14–20
  See also psychological processes
Leibniz, G. W., 52
Locke, John, 52
logos, 11

Maharshi, Ramana, 85
maṇḍala, 69, 76, 103
mantra, 3, 4, 18, 36, 37, 78, 91, 92
Manu, 13, 14, 36
meaning, 34, 38, 39, 67, 79
meditation, 58
memory, 51, 53, 54, 55, 57, 58, 59, 60, 91, 98
  memory and the unconscious, 63–64
mescaline, 67
Miller, Barbara, 42
Mīmāṁsā, 14
mind, 78
  as active, 52
  as passive, 52
  See also consciousness
mokṣa, 1, 4, 6, 22, 23, 24, 35, 36, 39, 40, 45, 91
motivation, 54, 55, 60, 91
Mumme, Patricia, 84
mysticism, 71–82, 89

nāda, 30
Nietzsche, 11, 20
Nirvāṇa, 2
niyamas, 36, 46–47

omniscience, 58, 59, 60, 64, 66, 83
Ornstein, Robert, 7, 88–89
Otto, Rudolf, 82

passion (*rāga*), 43, 44
Passmore, John, 89, 93
paśyanti vāk. *See vāk*
Patañjali, 11, 12, 17, 21, 36, 40, 43, 45, 46, 51, 52, 54, 56, 58, 59, 60, 61, 63, 64, 77, 78, 79, 80, 81, 82, 86, 89, 92
Pauli, Wolfgang, 65
perception, 12, 65–68, 80
  extra-sensory (ESP), 67
  supersensuous. *See pratibhā*
phoneme, 31
Plato, 58
pleasure as pain in the making, 44
prajñā, 25, 39, 40, 67, 68, 69
prakti, 15, 24, 95
prāṇa, 30, 34, 35, 37
prāṇāyāma, 37, 38, 39, 47
pratibhā, 1, 7, 39, 40, 65, 66, 67, 77
pratyahāra, 37, 38, 47
Pribram, Karl, 53, 55
psychological processes in speaking, 26–30
  in hearing, 30–35

Psychology, modern Western, 51, 83–92.
See also Freud, Jung, Pribram, Transpersonal
puruṣa, 15, 16, 19, 24, 52, 53, 95

Radhakrishnan, Sarvepali, 84
Raja, K. Kunjunni, 95
reincarnation, 58, 83, 89
See also saṁsāra
release from rebirth (salvation), 14, 19, 20
See also mokṣa
ritual prayer, 18
Roland, Alan, 7, 72
Ṛṣis, 13, 14, 16, 17, 18, 23, 36
Ryle, Gilbert, 62

śabda, 28, 30, 33, 34, 40, 79
Śabdabrahman, 22, 24, 35, 36, 39, 40
Śabdapūrvayoga, 22, 35, 39, 40
as interpreted by the *Yoga Sūtras*, 36–40
samādhi, 1, 2, 4, 18, 34, 38, 39, 40, 48, 78, 79, 81, 85, 89
nirvicāra samādhi, 3, 18, 19, 35, 40, 48, 78, 80, 82
nirvitarka samādhi, 18, 39, 80, 82
savicara samādhi, 19, 34, 35, 39, 40, 80, 82
savitarka samādhi, 18, 35, 39, 40, 79
saṁsāra, 1, 25, 45
saṁskāra, 1, 2, 22, 24, 25, 29, 31, 32, 33, 34, 35, 40, 51, 52, 53, 54, 57, 58, 59, 60, 63, 64, 65, 67, 68, 91
Śaṅkara, 12, 13, 14, 15, 16, 17, 19, 20
saṅketa, 33, 34, 35
Sāṅkhya-Yoga, 14, 20, 21, 24, 77, 84
Sastri, G., 22
self, 52, 53, 68, 69, 73, 74, 75, 76, 77, 81, 89
I-self, 7, 87
we-self, 7, 87
siddhis (psychic powers), 81
smṛti, 23
speaking, 26–30
sphoṭa, 24, 25, 26, 27, 29, 31, 32, 33, 34, 35, 36, 37, 38, 39, 40
śruti, 23
Stace, Walter, 71, 72, 77, 82
Stcherbatsky, T. H., 1
St. Paul, 75, 82
synapse, 54

tabula rasa (mind as), 52
Taoism, 77
Tart, Charles, 7, 88–89, 91
telepathy, 13
Transpersonal Psychology, 85ff., 91, 92

unconscious, 55, 56, 57, 58, 60, 63–64, 66, 67, 69, 73, 74, 75, 92
Upaniṣads, 84

Vairāgya-Śataba of Bhartṛhari, 42ff.
vāk, 23, 35, 36, 38, 39, 96
madhyamā vāk, 30, 35, 37, 38, 39, 40
paśyanti vāk, 25, 26, 37, 39
sūkmā vāk, 27
vaikhari vāk, 30, 33, 35, 37, 38, 39
Vākyapadīya of Bhartṛhari, 21, 22, 23, 24, 25, 26, 28, 30, 31, 33, 39, 95
Varenne, Jean, 83, 84
vāsanā, 15, 25, 36, 51, 52, 59, 91
Veda, 11, 14, 16, 18, 20, 21, 23, 26

Washburn, Michael, 7, 86–87
Wilbur, Ken, 86
Woodworth, Robert, 52

Yamas, 36, 46
Yoga, 1–5, 55, 56, 57, 58, 59, 82, 87, 89
Yoga and human nature, 83–90
Yoga and memory, 52–60
Yoga and modern Psychology, 61–63
Yoga and mysticism, 77–81, 89
Yoga and perception, 65–67
Yoga of the Word, 3, 36–40
Yoga techniques (*yogāṅga*), 36–39, 43, 46ff.
Yoga Sūtras of Patañjali, 1, 2, 5, 7, 11, 51, 56, 59, 61, 68, 78, 83, 84, 85, 89, 90, 91, 92, 95, 98–99
Yoga Sūtras assumed by Bhartṛhari, 21–40
Yoga Sūtras assumed in *Vairāgya- Śataka*, 42–48
Yoga Sūtras on language, 12–20

zen, 58, 67